Herbs for the Mind

WHAT SCIENCE
TELLS US ABOUT
NATURE'S
REMEDIES FOR

herbs *for the* mind

DEPRESSION,
STRESS, MEMORY
LOSS, AND
INSOMNIA

Jonathan R.T. Davidson, MD
Kathryn M. Connor, MD

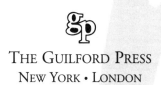

THE GUILFORD PRESS
NEW YORK • LONDON

© 2000 The Guilford Press
A Division of Guilford Publications, Inc.
72 Spring Street, New York, NY 10012
www.guilford.com

The information in this volume is not intended as a substitute for
consultation with healthcare professionals. Each individual's
health concerns should be evaluated by a qualified professional.

Printed in the United States of America

This book is printed on acid-free paper.

Last digit is print number: 9   8   7   6   5   4   3   2   1

Library of Congress Cataloging-in-Publication Data

Davidson, Jonathan R. T., 1943–
     Herbs for the mind : what science tells us about nature's
remedies for depression, stress, memory loss, and insomnia /
Jonathan R. T. Davidson, Kathryn M. Connor.
          p. cm.
     Includes bibliographical references and index.
     ISBN 1-57230-572-X (cloth) — ISBN 1-57230-476-6 (pbk.)
     1. Herbs—Therapeutic use.   2. Mental illness—Nutritional
aspects.   3. Neuropharmacology.   I. Connor, Kathryn M.   II.
Title.

RM666.H33 D378 2000
615'.78—dc21

                                                    00-026341

To Meg, Ben, and Becky,
and
Tom and Eleanor

Kinship is healing; we are physicians to each other.

—OLIVER SACKS, *Awakenings* (1973)

Contents

Acknowledgments

Herbs for the Mind grew out of a collaboration between the two of us that began about four years ago and is sustained and enriched by a wide range of shared interests and ideals. During the course of our collaboration, we discovered a common interest in herbal medicine and its potential to reduce the burden of emotional stress and psychological disorder in the many people who are so affected. At a time when few of our colleagues in conventional medicine thought the topic to be worth even a passing thought, we decided to embark on a program of research and study in this field, especially as it applies to our professional specialty of psychological medicine. We saw a need to bring together, as we hope we have done in this book, the existing information on major herbal remedies for psychological disorders as well as common daily problems, such as depression, stress, memory problems, and insomnia. To this information we wanted to add our joint experience as clinical practitioners, researchers, and teachers. Thus was born *Herbs for the Mind*.

Ultimately, many colleagues, friends, and family members have made this book possible, some in ways that are self-evident, others in more indirect ways. We would like to acknowledge debts of gratitude to the following individuals: Jacques Bradwejns, Donald Brown, Bernard Carroll, Jerry Cott, Peter Fisher, Susan Gaylord, Marianne Heger, Natalie Koether, Ranga Krishnan, Costas Loullis, David Reilly, David Riley, Jerilyn Ross, Richard Weisler, and Qun-Yi Zheng. It is extremely doubtful that this book would have ever seen the light of day if we had not had the good fortune to work with an exceptionally skilled clinical and research staff in the Anxiety and Traumatic Stress Program at Duke University. From them, we have learned that perhaps the most powerful drug comes in the form of the right word spoken, or the empathy of accurate and careful listening. It is through the right alliance that suffering is healed. On their own, the best drugs, the best herbs, the best psychotherapies, are all worth little.

Each of us, Jonathan and Kathy, wishes to express gratitude to our closest friends and family. Jonathan knows that this book would never have been written without the constant encouragement, support, and radiant good humor of his wife, Meg, over the years. His children have been important contributors to *Herbs for the Mind* as well. Ben served an invaluable role in providing ideas and information as we put the book together, and Becky brought her own very helpful insights to our work. From an early age, Jonathan has known where he wanted to sail his ship, and it has stayed true to course. For this he expresses gratitude to his parents, Kathleen and Robert, for giving him a home in which a strong sense of self was forged and opportunities always abounded. Collaborating on this book with Kathy has been a special joy, and has kept his creative energies in good supply. Whenever he has flagged, her drive, commitment, and focus has invariably put him back on track.

On another personal note, Kathy expresses gratitude to her family, whose love and support have been instrumental in helping her find and follow her star: to her parents, Tom and Eleanor, for instilling in her the skills to weather the storms and the faith to know that, though the course may vary, she will reach her destination; to her brother, Tom, for his encouragement and tactical prowess; and to Buck for his support, patience, and hand in steadying the course. She is also grateful to have had the privilege to work with and to learn from a wonderful mentor, respected colleague, and dear and special friend, Jonathan.

In conceptualizing, designing, and shaping the book, we are deeply indebted to the guidance and experience of Kitty Moore and Christine Benton, both of whom have helped to shape our original vision into a better one. Throughout the entire project, our administrative assistant, Sharon Lloyd, has been a tower of strength and great patience, as she has worked and reworked the manuscript through its various stages.

Introduction

He that will not apply new remedies must expect new
evils; for time is the great innovator.
> —SIR FRANCIS BACON, "Of Innovations,"
> *Essays* (1597–1625)

A disorder that requires no physician is preferable to any
that does.
> —HORACE WALPOLE, fourth Earl of Orford
> (1717–1797)

A phenomenon is unfolding in American health
care. It's no secret that alternative medical treatments are not so "alternative" anymore. Forty percent of Americans now
opt for some sort of nontraditional therapy for what ails them, and they
spend about $20 billion every year on these choices. Clearly, traditional
Western medicine does not satisfy all the health care needs of today's consumers. Perhaps more surprising, though, is the epidemic growth in popularity of herbs for the mind. More and more Americans are taking herbs to
soothe their psychological aches and pains, from depression to stress, from
insomnia to memory loss.

What accounts for the fact that ginkgo and St. John's wort, respectively, held the number-1 and number-2 slots among top-selling herbals in
the 1998 food, drug, and mass-merchandise market? How did kava's use
leap by 473 percent to become number 8 during that year? What brought
modest valerian to number 12 on that list?

1

Ask anyone you find mulling over the choices in a health food store why he is looking for an herbal remedy and you'll get a variety of answers. Use of herbal remedies in general has virtually exploded in the United States in the last few years. Herbal remedies are appealing options for many people with a holistic health orientation. For others, alternative therapies like herbs confer a sense of some control over one's destiny, which can be morale-building when one is coping with a serious illness. Still others turn to herbs as a result of growing dissatisfaction with more conventional forms of medical treatment. Perhaps the shopper you encounter has suffered intolerable side effects from a prescription drug or found its cost prohibitive or simply found it ineffective. Maybe anything labeled "natural" sounds safe and environmentally friendly. Possibly it's just easier to bypass the increasingly complex process of seeing a doctor to obtain a prescription, and opt instead to purchase something that doesn't require a prescription at all. Or maybe, like the rest of us, this shopper has been barraged with varied but always enthusiastic claims about the powers of certain herbs to rid us of what we view as some of society's most destructive ills: depression, stress, anxiety, insomnia, and mental decline.

Unfortunately, much of what consumers know about herbal remedies is riddled with myth and misinformation, or is at best incomplete. While sales of herbal products have increased at least fourfold during the 1990s, reliable facts about these preparations have not spread with the same wildfire speed. Many consumers today are taking herbal remedies incorrectly, denying themselves the very real benefits that *some* herbs offer. Some of us are taking the wrong herbs or the wrong combinations of herbs for the problems we have. A few of us may even be ignoring serious conditions that require medical attention. Then there are the die-hard skeptics, who view all herbal medicines—and, indeed, the raft of other alternative treatments coming into favor today—as nothing more than "snake oil." This last group appears, however, to belong to an ever-shrinking minority.

Possibly the greatest mystery embedded in the phenomenon of the booming herbal remedies market is the willingness of many consumers to ingest so-called dietary supplements extracted from plants without first getting answers to all of their questions about them. Ask the average herbal remedy shopper what is actually in that remedy he holds in his hand, and he probably won't be able to tell you. Ask if he knows whether there is any reliable scientific evidence that the product he's considering buying will do what he expects it to do, and the answer is likely to be "No." Ask why he considers "natural" products so benign and pharmaceutical products so suspect, and he will probably be at a loss to reply.

Prod the skeptics to tell you why they won't try any of these popular remedies, and they probably won't admit that sometimes "snake oil" turns out to have merit, even if it can't possibly do all it's claimed to do. The history of medicine is rife with examples of discoveries that were initially scoffed at and later applauded. In the 1800s, Dr. Ignaz Semmelweis, a Viennese physician, was ridiculed to the point of suffering an emotional breakdown when he suggested that many women were dying during childbirth simply because their doctors were not washing their hands. Today, of course, it is conventional wisdom that infections are caused by germs spread through unhygienic practices.

The truth is depression hurts, stress kills, anxiety is unnerving, insomnia is debilitating, and faulty memory is a major disadvantage in today's demanding world. The fact that these problems are viewed as so damaging to the quality of our lives today is one reason that herbs that apparently treat them are grouped together in this book. We are right to seek remedies for these disturbances of mind and body. If we can find help on the shelves of retail stores, saving the time and cost of a doctor's visit and a prescription, and simultaneously take a bit more control over the management of our own problems as part of our overall attempt at improved self-care, good for us. But woe be to those who seek the "quick fix" remedy without educating themselves thoroughly.

Marketed as "dietary supplements," herbal remedies are not regulated as stringently as medicines. This shortcoming leaves consumers somewhat unprotected by watchdogs like the U.S. Food and Drug Administration (FDA) and demands that we exercise extra caution in our choices of manufacturers, products, and forms of the remedies we intend to take. We also have to become avid but discriminating readers. Information on herbal remedies is constantly flowing forth, but not all of it is accurate or up to date. Finally, by joining the trend toward increasing self-care we shift some of the responsibility for reading our symptoms from our doctors to ourselves. Those who self-prescribe over-the-counter remedies of any kind must pay close attention to how they feel and how their symptoms change over time. If you find yourself unsure of whether anything is truly "wrong" and what to do about it, don't hesitate to see your doctor. Keep in mind that nagging symptoms that you may interpret as "the blues" or being "stressed out" or "tense" or "too wired to sleep" can be caused by medical problems that require professional attention.

Before treating yourself with *any* herbal remedy for *any* problem, know that there is no such thing as a fully safe treatment—"natural" herbal products most definitely included. Even placebos—inactive substances—have side effects, and it is unlikely that any active treatment could have fewer side effects than a placebo.

Are herbal remedies such as those covered in this book more environmentally friendly than manufactured medicines? This is debatable. It depends first on the conditions under which a plant has been grown, harvested, and conveyed from cultivator to distributor. Unscrupulous entrepreneurs do try to pass off immature and poorly cultivated crops, not to mention adulterated ones, as effective remedies. Finally, there is the potential for and serious threat of crop overdevelopment, with attendent risks of extinction of popular plant species.

This issue and many other philosophical points in the ongoing alternative-versus-traditional-medicine debate are beyond the scope of this book. Our goal is to fill you in on the latest information produced by laboratory and clinical research as well as by our combined experience in treating the common psychological problems that impair the daily lives of so many of us today. In these pages we share our own extensive professional experience as psychiatrists who have been treating patients in an academic medical setting at Duke University Medical Center. This setting has given us an outstanding opportunity to provide care to a very wide range of psychiatric patients, especially those suffering from depression, anxiety, and stress. It has also afforded us many opportunities to conduct research into discovering new treatments as well as to provide teaching and supervision to our colleagues in training. In the last few years, we have found that herbal remedies can be integrated usefully into patient care and we now use them at times in regular treatment, as well as in the research setting.

We became interested in herbal remedies about three or four years ago, as an outgrowth of a more general interest in complementary treatments. Earlier, for example, one of us had undertaken personal training and research in homeopathic medicine. Seeing herbal medicine as a field of great importance to medical practice spurred us to conduct some research into this field of practice. We conducted a survey of the uses of herbal and other complementary treatments in our patients. We also began a study of kava for that treatment of generalized anxiety. At that time we sensed that few people possessed reliable information about herbal remedies but that most were open-minded and wanted to know more. Most of their information, for better or worse, was gleaned from the popular media and/or the Internet.

We believe you deserve to know exactly what is in the remedies you take and to be given adequate information about the products you're considering purchasing. We think you should know how much reliable scientific evidence has been gathered regarding whether St. John's wort can ease depression, whether kava can alleviate stress and anxiety, whether ginkgo can slow the rate of declining memory in those with dementing illness, and whether valerian can help you get the sleep you need. And we think you should understand exactly how to get the best positive effect from these remedies with the fewest possible side effects.

The following four chapters include all of that information. But, as discriminating consumers and managers of your own health, you will want to know a lot more. What the weekly magazines, TV talk shows, and your best friend won't or can't tell you includes not only the therapeutic limitations of these herbs but also their lesser known benefits. Ginkgo, for example, may not be the "fountain of youth" it's touted to be, but did you know it is used successfully to reverse the sexual dysfunction that is a common side effect of drugs like Prozac? St. John's wort hasn't been shown to be a panacea for all psychological ills, as some of its advocates claim, but it has an active effect on a wide range of neurochemicals in the brain and may prove to have even more varied effects than you've been reading about elsewhere. Sure, kava makes many people feel nice and relaxed, and it's no surprise that it's served in "bars," not only in Polynesia but increasingly in the United States too. But when taken judiciously, it not only relieves stress but actually sharpens the wits—unlike alcohol and other recreational drugs. Then there's valerian, a well-established sleep aid but also a potential help for many people who suffer from stress and mild anxiety. The point is that some claims about these herbs are exaggerated, but other benefits they can confer are virtually ignored. We'll fill you in on all of this.

On the other side of the coin, reports that herbal remedies are completely safe and benign leave a lot unsaid that you should hear. Scientific investigation into herbal remedies is a new field of endeavor in the United States. Thus most of our data come from investigations conducted in Europe. However, we have almost no data from anywhere about the long-term use of these four herbs. It may actually be perfectly safe to take St. John's wort, ginkgo, kava, or valerian for several years, but we don't know for sure yet. Nor do we know whether taking one of these herbs in the short term will have any undesirable consequences further into the future, though indications so far are that they will not. This is the type of information you need to have to make an informed decision about when and how to use one of these self-help remedies. This is the type of information you will find throughout this book.

Along the same lines, these herbs seem to have very few side effects when used judiciously and in the short term. But it's important to understand that for the herbs discussed in this book we have nothing as precise as the numerical data we have concerning the adverse effects of pharmaceutical agents. So although signs are good, it is important to keep in mind that the data are limited and that there is still much to be learned.

It is, in fact, just as important to know which questions can't be answered yet as it is to know where hard data exist. We should remember that while many positive outcome studies are published, those studies that find a treatment to be *ineffective* do not always get into print. Throughout this book we will tell you what scientists still don't understand about the four herbs discussed, what issues need to be investigated further, and what new information you can expect to become available in the years ahead. Those we treat have taught us a lot about the typical concerns of people who treat their psychological problems with herbs. In every chapter we pose the questions most often asked in our offices, and provide the answers we give to our patients—including "We just don't know yet" when that is the case. To us, this constant exchange of information is an example of the therapeutic alliance between doctor and patient at its best.

Many of you have undoubtedly rejected the outdated no-questions-asked, always-bow-to-authority mode of doctor–patient relationships, and with good reason. But please don't deny yourself the benefits of professional medical advice altogether. When in doubt, always call your doctor. Throughout this book we have inserted caveats about when you should consider seeing a doctor rather than self-treating with herbs; when you *must*, for the sake of your health, take herbs only under a doctor's supervision; and when you should not take these herbs at all. Though horror stories abound about the dire consequences that have befallen some individuals who have relied on herbal products, most of these tragedies have been attributed either to poor-quality, tainted products or to extreme misuse or abuse of the products. But there is always risk in taking any medicine, including medicinal herbs, and the more severe your medical problems, the more cautious you should be in self-treating any symptoms of any kind.

It is not the intention of this book to encourage you to diagnose yourself, especially if you have a mental or emotional condition that signifi-

*cantly impairs your life. Diagnosis is the job of qualified medical profes-
sionals. Throughout this book you will find guidelines for assessing the
possible severity of your psychological symptoms, with warnings about
consulting a doctor whenever professional help may be necessary.*

Nor is it our intention to oversell any of the herbal remedies in this
book. At times as you read you may get the impression that these herbs *are*
in fact "miracle drugs." We can't deny that we are excited—as researchers
looking at the effects of these plant extracts and as clinicians treating real
people with real problems—about the potential for these herbs to ease debilitating symptoms suffered by millions of adults around the world. But
please take our warnings as seriously as our enthusiasm. The amount of research evidence amassed for these remedies represents a fraction of the evidence we have concerning all aspects of prescription and over-the-counter
pharmaceuticals. *We have a lot more to learn.* And remember that the "placebo response" can be potent for any disorder: *Don't be overtaken by the
power of suggestion.*

These caveats aside, the information you'll find in this book represents
the views and experience of two professionals who are very well versed in
scientific and clinical medicine, and who have also received training in
complementary and alternative medicine. A number of excellent books
have been published on St. John's wort, ginkgo, kava, or valerian alone.
Many other books touch on these herbal remedies as a part of a broader
canvas. Our book is designed to provide a balanced and in-depth account
of herbs that treat depression, anxiety, stress, aging and memory problems,
and insomnia—herbs whose use is on the rise.

A Brief History:
Herbs for the Mind as Alternative Medicine

Until the early 1990s in the United States, herbs for the mind were really
the domain of a small number of freethinking or unusually health-aware
people. The great mass of people paid little attention to such forms of treatment. Thus the herbs we discuss in this book were limited pretty much to
the shelves of small health food stores. Today, of course, all of that has
changed. Not only are these herbal preparations and many more available
in supermarkets, but physicians trained in traditional Western medicine are
becoming better informed on the use of herbs and other alternative treatments—in large part because their patients are demanding it.

Anyone who travels outside the United States or who has ties to other cultures knows that the use of herbal remedies and other alternative treatments for physical and emotional problems has a long history extending back to antiquity. In fact, in the rest of the world alternative treatments are still widely used today, often side by side with modern medical practices. In 1993, the World Health Organization (WHO) estimated that 80 percent of the world's population received primary health care through traditional medicine, herbs, and medicinal plants.

Interest in complementary and alternative medicine (CAM), including herbal remedies, in the United States has lagged behind such interest in the rest of the world. But in the last 10 years the use of CAM in the United States has grown considerably: a survey in 1990 showed that 34 percent of Americans had used some form of alternative therapy in the preceding year, a figure that increased to 42 percent by 1997. One of the areas enjoying the greatest growth in popularity was herbal medicine. In 1994 the total U.S. sales of herbal products amounted to $1.6 billion; and by 1998 sales exceeded $4 billion. Sales may well surpass $6 billion in 1999, a figure already achieved in the European marketplace. This is truly big business! A large proportion of these revenues includes the sale of herbs that help to treat common emotional disturbances, such as depression and anxiety, as well as insomnia and memory problems.

When we began exploring the use of herbal remedies, most of our colleagues remained unimpressed, silently wondering why we did not make better use of our time or even why we would risk harming our own careers (a prophecy that fortunately does not seem to have come true). The majority of our patients, on the other hand, drew comfort from knowing that they had found professionals who were prepared to listen noncritically and even to be supportive of their own hopes and views about taking herbal remedies. Some patients, of course, were not very responsive when we suggested that they consider an herbal approach. That was fine, too, since we had no desire to impose our views on those who had other convictions.

Today the climate is changing, and many medical schools are now offering courses on herbal and other alternative treatments. At Duke University, for instance, there is a strong program of this type, under the direction of our colleague in radiology, Dr. Larry Burk. It is well attended and has drawn Duke and community practitioners together. While most MDs throughout the country are still perhaps reluctant to initiate and/or prescribe herbal treatments, they are in general more open-minded and better informed than in the past.

The historical reluctance of American consumers and health care practitioners to rely on what they often viewed as less sophisticated folk medicine has to do with the almost miraculous advances we have witnessed in Western medicine over the last 50 years. Newer, we have been prone to believe, is usually better. Fortunately, Americans are now beginning to realize that "folk" remedies that have been accepted in many cultures for thousands of years probably have some good reasons for surviving. Not everything that springs from the earth is sold by snake oil salesmen or destined for a witches' brew. Ironically, many people today are unaware that some of our most valuable medicines come to us from plants. Most of us are familiar with the more notorious examples: cocaine from the tropical coca plant and morphine and heroin from the opium poppy. But how many people know that willow bark gives us aspirin, foxglove provides the digitalis for heart patients, and other plants are the sources of malaria-fighting quinine and the decongestant pseudoephedrine? And the list goes on.

Americans are only now learning what Europeans and Asians have known for a long time. St. John's wort and *Ginkgo biloba*, for example, have been widely used in Germany and France for generations and are now among the most widely prescribed medicines in those countries. Forms of treatment that we in the United States (as well as in some other parts of the West) consider unorthodox, such as homoeopathy and herbal medicine, have always been more widely accepted in Central Europe. Recently, the use of herbal remedies in medicine received a big boost thanks to the German health care system, which not only endorses such treatments but also commissioned a group of experts to critically review the data on herbal products.

The German government established a regulatory body called Commission E (similar to the U.S. FDA) to review data pertaining to the safety and efficacy of herbs. Based on these evaluations, Commission E approves or disapproves specific standardized herbal treatments and provides recommendations for their use accordingly. The commission's findings have been published in a compendium called the German Commission E Monographs. This authoritative text, recently translated into English, has been the most popular book in the herbal marketplace during 1999. Commission E's report on the effectiveness and safety of these treatments has been used to determine indications for many herbal treatments, which are as a result well integrated into the health care system. You will read about Commission E's findings throughout this book.

Another popular herbal resource is the *Physicians' Desk Reference for*

Herbal Medicines (or *Herbal PDR*). This book contains information similar to that found in the German Commission E Monographs. The *Herbal PDR* is organized like the *Physicians' Desk Reference* for prescription medications, a popular physician's resource that can be found in most doctors' offices across the United States. Therefore, the format used in the *Herbal PDR* is very familiar to U.S. physicians, which makes it easy for them to use.

In a published study by our group at Duke, over 40 percent of patients seeing us for anxiety or depression reported that they had used some form of complementary or alternative treatment for either their emotional or their physical health in the previous year. The following four chapters discuss the most frequently used and best studied herbal treatments for emotional and psychological problems today, but they are certainly not your only treatment options.

Take depression as an example. Other popular and/or effective treatments for managing depression could include S-adenosylmethionine (SAMe), a natural substance present in the body that has been shown in a number of clinical studies to help people with depression. This treatment is well tolerated and has few side effects. However, SAMe is not an herbal treatment and therefore falls outside the scope of this book. The same is true of 5-HTP (5-hydroxytryptophan), a precursor natural substance that the body turns into the neurochemical serotonin. Acupuncture is yet another treatment recently found effective for depression, according to studies conducted at the University of Arizona. However, this is not a self-administered treatment, and qualified acupuncturists are in short supply at the present time.

Other kinds of alternative treatments for depression, anxiety, stress, and insomnia include meditation, chiropractic, and homeopathy. We recently conducted a small uncontrolled study that found lowering of depression and anxiety associated with the use of different homeopathic remedies. Except for SAMe in depression and phosphatidyl serine in memory impairment, the effectiveness of alternative treatments for the problems addressed in this book is less well established. Still, you may find that these treatments relieve some of your distress. In our survey, meditational, spiritual, and herbal treatments were the most commonly reported treatment options, in that order. Most of those who had used these approaches reported that they felt the treatments had been helpful, and that when they used them, they tended to do so repeatedly.

To find out more about these various alternatives, we recommend that you consult the various books available or discuss the treatments with a specialist in that particular field. Two books that we have found useful are *Alternative Medicine: What Works: A Comprehensive, Easy-to-Read Review of the Scientific Evidence, Pro and Con*, by Adriane Fugh-Berman, MD, published by Williams and Wilkins (1997), and *Dr. Rosenfeld's Guide to Alternative Medicine: What Works, What Doesn't, and What's Right for You*, published by Random House (1999).

Other herbs that have traditionally been used for depression include ginkgo and kava; for stress and anxiety, passionflower, reishi, and hops have been advocated; for memory problems, sage, huperzine, and peony; and for sleep, chamomile, lemon balm, passionflower, and kava. However, there has been practically no research in these areas to date.

How Herbs Get into Stores: Government Regulations and Manufacturers' Standards

The explosive growth of the herbal market has created something of a monster run amok in the United States. With the potential for profits seemingly endless, more and more companies are jumping on the herbal bandwagon, adding more products to a vast market that is essentially operating without government oversight and regulation. This growth raises important concerns about quality control.

In the United States a number of steps were taken in the early 1990s to address these concerns. Before 1994, if an herbal product was suspected of causing harm, the FDA could order the manufacturer to withdraw its product until the manufacturer had proven it to be safe. The onus was placed on the manufacturer. To many, this made the costs of introducing new herbal products prohibitive. Then, in 1994, Congress passed the Dietary Supplement Health and Education Act (DSHEA), which was designed to transfer the responsibility for proving harm to the FDA. Consequently DSHEA encouraged the introduction of many more dietary supplements.

But the act was not without problems. DSHEA prohibited a manufacturer from making any claims that a dietary supplement can treat a disease but allowed claims that a supplement could enhance structure or function. This means that the label on a St. John's wort package could not say that the herb helps to treat depression. Instead, you'd see vague claims for various benefits such as "central nervous system health." For an herb that had laxative properties, its effect would probably be quite clear, because the label would be allowed to state that the product "promotes regularity" even though it would not be permitted to say it "cures constipation." But for psychological disturbances, which may produce a variety of less straightforward symptoms, phrases like "promotes healthy emotional balance" can certainly mean a variety of things. Needless to say, consumers cannot depend on labels alone when they are looking for the right product for their symptoms. Furthermore, these vague statements may contribute to the misconception that herbs like St. John's wort heal *everything* that ails us psychologically.

Critics of DSHEA are also concerned about the general lack of regulations governing dietary supplements in the United States. Any business that wants to market a drug for the treatment of a disease (including depression, anxiety, insomnia, and dementia) must undergo a long, rigorous, and costly test process under the stipulations of the Food, Drug and Cosmetics Act (FDCA), which set the standards for drug development. Such a test program can cost a pharmaceutical company well over $100 million. Few herbal companies are in a position to invest this kind of money, particularly since there is limited patent protection on herbal products. It is interesting that a number of the major pharmaceutical houses are now turning their sights toward herbal products, perhaps in acknowledgment of the growing market, among other reasons. These include (but are not limited to) Warner–Lambert, American Home Products, SmithKline Beecham, Bayer, and Novartis. Thanks to the huge advertising budgets they have at their disposal, we can expect market penetrance of herbal products to become even bigger. We hope, too, that these deep pockets will support the high-quality research that needs to be done.

DSHEA may ultimately be modified even further over time. Built into the act was a call for a commission on dietary supplement labels to review the definition of disease and assess good manufacturing standards. This commission met and gave its report to the FDA during 1998; its results were published in January 2000.

In response to input from industry and the public, the FDA expanded the number of acceptable structure/function claims, revising the definition of disease. Structure/function claims are now permitted for common, but nonserious, symptoms associated with adolescence, pregnancy, menopause, and aging. A product such as black cohosh, for example, could previously carry a label with a vague claim such as "promotes health in postmenopausal women." Now it is acceptable to claim that it "treats (the symptom of) hot flashes." A product such as ginkgo, for example, could now claim to treat "mild memory loss associated with aging," but not the disease of dementia. Of course, this still leaves some doubt as to how a person could distinguish between normal age-related memory loss and the onset of a more serious dementia. Full details of the FDA's statement can be found at http://vm.cfsan.fda.gov.

For now, there are basically four ways in which an herbal remedy can be introduced to the U.S. consumer market: (1) as a food, such as ginger root or hot red pepper; (2) as an herbal/dietary supplement; (3) as an over-the-counter medication; or (4) as a prescription drug. If a company wishes to market a product as a dietary supplement, then it must be in compliance with DSHEA. If a company wishes to develop and market a drug, then it must comply with the stricter and much more expensive provisions of the FDCA.

The FDA is prepared to challenge a manufacturer if the agency believes that a dietary supplement is in fact a drug. A recent case involved Cholestin, a dietary supplement derived from red yeast rice, which has long been used in traditional Chinese medicine to promote blood circulation. Cholestin, which lowers cholesterol, contains lovastatin, a compound present in successfully marketed drugs for lowering cholesterol, such as Mevacor. The FDA held that Cholestin was really a drug that should not be sold under the guise of a dietary supplement, and therefore attempted to ban the product. According to the FDA, the manufacturer would either have to stop selling Cholestin or carry out an elaborate and costly series of studies to show that it worked and was safe under the rules of the FDCA. After a lengthy legal struggle in federal court, a judge ruled that Cholestin was not a drug but a dietary supplement and could continue to be sold as such. In this case the FDA had to eat humble pie. We can probably expect many similar disputes in the future.

Meanwhile, as the FDA and manufacturers battle over such designations, we consumers still have little way of knowing exactly what is in many of the herbal products that hit the shelves. The standards for manufacturing, marketing, and labeling of so-called dietary supplements are far less stringent than those required for over-the-counter medicine, prescription drugs, and even food. Tests done on broad samples of different herbal products have resulted in some alarming discoveries: for example, some supplements contain much less (even none) of the claimed active ingredient, while other remedies are tainted by harmful ingredients.

As you'll read in the following chapters, the best benchmark of efficacy is standardization of the active ingredient. If the label says the product contains a "standardized extract," the product contains a certain percentage of the active ingredient so that you know how much of that ingredient, by weight, is in your daily dose. The term *standardization* actually refers to the whole process by which the herb is chemically analyzed and guaranteed to have a certain content of a specific (supposedly) active ingredient, following stringent manufacturing specifications. These processes ensure consistency from one batch to the next. In each chapter we tell you what to look for in standardization.

A Concise Buyer's Guide: Shopping Tips and Consumer Safeguards

Besides looking for standardization, you can take other measures to increase your chances of buying a good-quality herbal preparation, *though there are still no guarantees of the kind you would expect with a prescription drug or even many over-the-counter remedies.*

You can start before heading out to the store by gathering general information about the manufacturers. The American Botanical Council at 1-800-373-7105 as well as on the World Wide Web at abc@herbalgram.org and www.herbalgram.org is a good resource. The American Botanical Council provides a most useful abstracting service that reviews the major developments concerning the herbal industry, and this is available by subscription.

There are many places to buy herbal products, including traditional pharmacies, grocery stores, large discount stores, health food stores, and even convenience stores. Mail order is another option. We do not have particular views about one or the other type of outlet but would rather emphasize the importance of carefully examining the product label, as we discuss below.

With the rapidly growing field of herbal products available in the dietary supplement market, shopping for the right supplement can be quite overwhelming. There are so many products to choose from! Which product should you buy? Should you try a dried extract in a pill or capsule, or perhaps a tea or a liquid tincture? What would be better, a single herb or a product containing a combination of herbs? What dose should you take and how often?

You will find that herbal products come in a variety of preparations. For instance, there are bulk herbs, which are sold much as they occur in nature—for example, garlic cloves or peppermint leaves. These bulk herbs may be steeped in boiling water to produce a tea called an "infusion," or ground into a fine powder for packaging in capsules or tablets. The potency and quality of these herbs vary widely, as you can imagine, and in this form are considered an unreliable way to get an effective dose of active herbal ingredients. An alternative to bulk herbs is a concentrated preparation of the whole herb, called an "extract." Extracts come in three forms:

- *Tinctures*: the mildest form of extract, prepared by soaking the herb in water or alcohol and pressing out the solution. The strength of the tincture is measured by its herb:solvent concentration, commonly a 1:5 ratio whereby it contains five times as much solvent as herbal product. Tinctures are generally less economical than other extract forms because of the large proportion of solvent.
- *Fluid extracts*: produced by evaporating the solvent to yield a 1:1 herb:solvent ratio. These are generally five times as strong as tinctures made from the same solution.
- *Solid extracts*: the solvent is completely removed, further concentrating the herbal material. Their strength is measured by the amount of crude extract used in their preparation, whereby a 4:1 concentration indicates that 4 grams of the crude herb was required to produce 1 gram of the solid extract. These formulations have the greatest chemical stability and are generally the most cost effective.

Here are a number of other tips and safeguards to help you in selecting and shopping for an herbal product:

Shopping Tips

- Read all labels carefully!
- Use single, whole-herb preparations when possible, since some herbs may well have several active constituents that act synergistically. As you'll read in the following chapters, very few reliable studies have looked at combination herb products, so you can't be sure of all the effects they may have. With a few exceptions noted in the chapters, we suggest you stick with the single-herb preparations for each of the herbs we review.
- Check the expiration date. If no expiration date is listed, put the bottle or box back on the shelf and pick another one.
- Do not make your selection based on price alone because an inexpensive product is not always a bargain. On the other hand, the most expensive products are not always the best either. Bottom line: read the label!

- Manufacturers' dosage guidelines vary widely and are not always based on information found in the scientific literature or in clinical practice. In the following chapters, we provide recommendations for daily dosing, duration of use, potential drug interactions, and other cautions when using herbs for the mind.

A Few Warnings for Everyone

- Are you pregnant, nursing, or thinking about conceiving? If your answer is Yes, you should first consult your doctor before taking a dietary supplement, or any over-the-counter or prescription medication.
- Do you have any medical problems for which you are (or should be) under the care of a physician, and/or are you taking any medications regularly for a medical condition? If your answer is Yes to either question, you should also consult your physician before using a dietary supplement.
- If you have a history of alcohol or drug problems, you should avoid tincture preparations, since they generally have a large alcohol content.
- When you do see your physician, be sure to inform him or her of any and all dietary supplements you are taking. Such information may impact on other medications your doctor may prescribe for you and may also help in diagnosing problems you may be having.
- Be alert for potential side effects and interactions.
- Follow label recommendations regarding any specific cautions and pertaining to potential interactions with alcohol or other drugs. Herbs can take time to work, so be patient if you do not note an effect immediately. Also, if a product seems to be helping you, more of the herb will not necessarily make you feel even better! A major cause of adverse reactions with herbal preparations is inappropriate use of the product by the consumer.

The Modern Therapeutic Alliance: Finding a Doctor Who Is Open to Herbal Remedies

Chapters 1 to 4 each contain information to help you determine whether you should be under a doctor's supervision while you take an herb. If you fall into any of these categories or if you are already seeing a doctor for the psychological problems covered in this book, how do you make sure your therapeutic alliance is formed with someone who is inclined or at least open to alternative therapies such as herbs? You may have to do a little work to find the right doctor, but you may be pleasantly surprised and discover that your present doctor is receptive to exploring these alternative treatment options.

Some conventionally trained doctors do use herbal and other complementary treatments in their practice: such doctors usually identify themselves by saying that they practice holistic medicine. Other health practitioners who use herbal remedies much more extensively include naturopaths, homeopaths, midwives, acupuncturists, physicians' associates, and practitioners of traditional Chinese medicine. If you are thinking about seeing such a practitioner, be sure to do your homework first and find a highly recommended individual.

One way to determine whether a doctor you are considering consulting is knowledgeable is by word of mouth from other patients from his or her practice. Also, openly ask the doctor about his or her knowledge and interests. Has the doctor had any previous experience using herbal remedies with his or her own patients? Has the doctor known of friends or relatives who have responded well to such treatments? This type of question is a good way to discover not only the doctor's experience but also his or her attitude toward alternative treatments in general.

Remember: treatment is not only about understanding the disorder you have, but also about understanding the person with the disorder. The best doctor is therefore the one who can treat your problems well and understand you equally well. At least one study has shown this therapeutic alliance to be more important to recovery than the specific type of treatment. A good way to find the right doctor for you is by referral from a friend, family member, colleague, or other person you respect. Another approach if you are depressed, for example, might be to contact your local depression support group or the National Manic-Depressive Association for specialists in the area. See the "Resources" section at the back of this book for additional information.

Don't assume that just because your current doctor has never suggested herbal remedies he or she is closed to the idea. A recent survey found that more than 80 percent of health practitioners wanted to learn more about herbal remedies, and between 40 and 60 percent felt that their knowledge needed to be increased. Again, alternative medicine is being offered more and more because of patient demand for it. Many doctors are open to encouragement in this direction from their patients.

A Word on Costs of Herbs for the Mind

In this book we do not recommend any specific brands or products. Brands are constantly being introduced or reformulated in a growing market, and for many of them sound clinical and safety data may not be available. While, in certain cases, specific brands have been found to be effective for particular disorders, and we can reaffirm such findings, we do not recommend specific brands or products. We do, however, include a survey that we have made of the products available for each herb toward the end of each chapter. The table summarizing the survey gives you an idea of how much products vary. Cost, as you will see, is one big variable, although the cost of herbals is sometimes low compared to the cost of a proprietary (nongeneric) drug.

Nevertheless, some people might find the cost prohibitive. Does health insurance cover herbal remedies? So far, most health insurance companies are just beginning to provide some coverage for alternative therapies, including homeopathy, naturopathy, herbal consultations, and Chinese herbal medicine, in addition to nonmedicinal treatments such as massage, reflexology, and biofeedback. At this time, it would be unusual for herbal remedies to be covered, any more than vitamins are. We do not know to what extent this could change.

How to Use This Book

Each of the following chapters is devoted to one of the principal herbs for the mind: St. John's wort, kava, ginkgo, and valerian. If you're sure what your problem is, read the appropriate chapter first: Chapter 1 for depression, Chapter 2 for stress and anxiety, Chapter 3 for memory impairment and age-related changes, and Chapter 4 for insomnia. But remember that (1) you may have misdiagnosed your own symptoms and (2) each of these herbs has more than one beneficial effect. So we strongly encourage you to read the whole book if you are interested in improving your psychological well-being as part of your general self-care. If you're not sure how your symptoms might be categorized, look for the lists of symptoms for each disturbance in each chapter and find the one that fits you most closely.

Each chapter is divided into three main sections, which address what the herb does, how it works, and how to use it. You'll want to read all three to be a well-informed consumer of these self-help remedies.

For more information, turn to the Resources and References sections at the back of the book. And, of course, remember that your health care professionals are one of the best resources you have.

1

St. John's Wort

The Herb of Light

There is no duty we so much underrate as the duty of
being happy.

—ROBERT LOUIS STEVENSON,
Virginibus Puerisque (1881)

The physicians of ancient Greece named it
Hyperikon, for "over an image [of a god]." The
medieval French called it *tutsan*, or "heals-all." For centuries what the English named *St. John's wort* has been used to cure all manner of ills, from wounds incurred in holy wars to snake bites to demonic possession. Today it is marketed in the United States as a "dietary supplement," and labels claim it can do everything from enhancing and balancing mood to promoting a positive mental outlook and a healthy central nervous system.

Popular press reports in the late 1990s sent Americans running to stores to find out for themselves whether St. John's wort is a miracle drug for the new millennium, a panacea for all of our emotional ailments. The "herb of light" enjoyed the fastest growing sale of any herb sold in the United States in 1998, and ranked number 2 in sales of all herbal remedies that year.

Eventually St. John's wort led the charge of herbal remedies from health food stores into supermarkets, where they now occupy a permanent place on well-shopped shelves. But being able to buy a bottle of St. John's wort along with a quart of milk and a loaf of bread has not made it the medicine-cabinet equivalent of aspirin or cold medicine. Consumers who eagerly purchased St. John's wort realized when they returned home that the package fell woefully short of answering their questions about its use.

Does its availability "over the counter" mean that St. John's wort is completely safe? Had they bought the best brand—or are all brands the same? Were the directions for taking it appropriate for everyone? How would they know it was working? For that matter, since different brands claimed different benefits, what benefits could consumers reasonably expect? Should the whole family take St. John's wort, like they did vitamins? Would it have any side effects? Could anyone become addicted to it? Could it be taken along with prescription medicines? Could it be taken if one was pregnant?

Answers to many of these questions are just beginning to emerge. Much of what has been reported as fact in magazines and on talk shows, by health food store clerks and on the Internet, has been based on anecdotal evidence or limited research investigations. In contrast, the information on safe and effective use of St. John's wort that you'll find in this chapter is based on scientific studies published through mid-1999, including placebo-controlled clinical trials, case reports, and studies on mechanism of action, that were conducted using sound research methods.

❦ WHAT ST. JOHN'S WORT DOES

Cliff, age 41, had not been feeling quite himself for several months. He still went to work, did his job, and participated in all the normal family activities, but not with his usual relish. He just couldn't seem to shake his recent feeling of sadness and accompanying low energy.

Brad, 27, had always had a short fuse. Now starting his third job in three years, he knew he couldn't afford to alienate his newest boss. But he was already snapping at his coworkers, and he found himself eating nothing all day and then stuffing himself once he got home, sleeping poorly, and struggling throughout each morning to focus on the reports that were starting to form a precarious pile on his desk.

Jackie, 18, seemed to change overnight—at least from her mother's point of view. Always an outgoing, cheerful child, she had started spending all her time locked in her room, sleeping into the middle of the afternoon on weekends. When confronted about the homework she couldn't seem to finish on time and the falling grades that resulted, all Jackie would say was "What's the point? Everybody's smarter than me anyway."

A Natural Antidepressant

Will St. John's wort lift Cliff's spirits, soothe Brad's irritability, and boost Jackie's self-esteem? It just might, but not because it is a cure-all. It might help because all of these problems are associated with depression, and St. John's wort is first and foremost an antidepressant.

Most of us are unaware of how broad-ranging the symptoms of depression are. It's easy to misinterpret poor eating and sleeping patterns, low energy, and difficulty concentrating as the widely familiar signs of stress when they may actually indicate clinical depression. In truth, if you have several of the following symptoms, you may be suffering from depression and thus may benefit from treatment with an antidepressant, including St. John's wort:

- Feeling sad or tearful
- Feeling hopeless about the future
- Being low in energy
- Sleeping poorly
- Sleeping too much
- Having poor appetite
- Having excess appetite
- Feeling worthless or guilty
- Concentrating poorly
- Forming ideas or plans about suicide

The accepted forms of treatment for depression today are medicine and psychotherapy. Antidepressants are the treatment of choice in most medical settings. You probably already know something about the class of drugs called *antidepressants*. Books like Peter Kramer's *Listening to Prozac*, as well as numerous articles and talk shows, have made Prozac and similar drugs collectively known as *selective serotonin reuptake inhibiting antidepressants* (SSRIs) household words. These more recent entries into the antidepressant arsenal are, however, only one of five main groups of medications developed to treat depression (see Table 1).

The older tricyclic drugs, introduced into psychiatry in the 1950s and

1960s, and the other older generation antidepressants—the monoamine oxidase inhibitor (MAOI) drugs, and the stimulants such as Dexedrine (dextroamphetamine) and Ritalin (methylphenidate)—are used less often in treating depression these days. The stimulants, however, are still often used to treat children with attention-deficit/hyperactivity disorder.

Table 1 lists St. John's wort by itself in the herbal category because it is the best known and most solidly established of the herbal or "natural" treatments for depression. Other herbs, such as kava (discussed in Chapter 2), are also used for depression, but we have less evidence indicating that they are truly effective. Other prescription drugs as well are sometimes used to treat depression, but usually only for very severe depression or as mood stabilizers, so they are not really comparable to the antidepressants.

Is St. John's wort essentially just another antidepressant that happens to grow naturally in the wild?

Not exactly. As Table 1 indicates, St. John's wort affects a large number of the chemicals found in the human brain. This may be a natural result of its being a complex botanical organism rather than a single chemical developed by a manufacturer: it may be that St. John's wort has more complicated, varied effects than the manufactured antidepressants. (However, although a "single-chemical" antidepressant may seem to have a straightforward mechanism of action, the truth is that we really do not know exactly how drugs such as Prozac work.) Although we don't know exactly what mechanism is responsible, the unique makeup of St. John's wort results in fewer side effects than at least the older antidepressants, against which it has been most frequently tested to date.

All these factors combine to make St. John's wort a major contender for treating at least mild forms of depression. While much more research needs to be done to determine the full scope of the herb's benefits and limitations, it's not surprising that St. John's wort's appeal has spread rapidly by word of mouth. Market research that identifies exactly who is buying over-the-counter St. John's wort preparations today, why they are buying them, and what benefits they are experiencing has yet to be done. But research and our own clinical experience strongly suggest that consumers are finding St. John's wort a readily obtainable, benign, and effective mild antidepressant—whether they were aware that the problems they are self-treating could be defined as depression or not.

Not all antidepressants will be effective in all cases, which is one reason

Table 1. Doses and Names of Main Antidepressant Medications

Generic name	Brand name	Daily dose (mg per day)	Presumed chemical action
Selective serotonin reuptake inhibitors			
Fluoxetine	Prozac	10–80	Serotonin
Sertraline	Zoloft	50–200	Serotonin
Paroxetine	Paxil	10–60	Serotonin
Fluvoxamine	Luvox	50–300	Serotonin
Citalopram	Celexa	20–60	Serotonin
Other new-generation drugs			
Venlafaxine	Effexor	37.5–375	Serotonin, noradrenaline[a]
Bupropion	Wellbutrin, Zyban	100–450	Noradrenaline, dopamine
Nefazodone	Serzone	150–600	Serotonin
Mirtazapine	Remeron	15–60	Serotonin, noradrenaline
Tricyclics			
Imipramine	Tofranil	25–300	Serotonin, noradrenaline
Amitriptyline	Elavil	25–300	Serotonin, noradrenaline
Doxepin	Sinequan	25–300	Serotonin, noradrenaline
Clomipramine	Anafranil	25–250	Serotonin
Desipramine	Pertofrane, Norpramine	25–300	Noradrenaline
Nortriptyline	Pamelor, Aventyl	25–200	Noradrenaline, serotonin
Trimipramine	Surmontyl	15–300	Noradrenaline
Protriptyline	Vivactil	10–60	Norepinephrine, serotonin
Others			
Phenelzine	Nardil	15–90	Serotonin, noradrenaline, dopamine
Tranylcypromine	Parnate	10–60	Serotonin, noradrenaline, dopamine
Herbal			
St. John's wort	Kira et al.	600–1,800	Serotonin, noradrenaline, dopamine, GABA, interleukin-6

[a]Also referred to in the United States as norepinephrine.

so much research and development has been devoted to the search for new antidepressants. No treatment works 100 percent of the time; indeed, a realistic expectation might be that any particular medicine has about a 70 percent chance of helping you. If the first medicine you try does not help you, there is a good chance that a second or third medicine will be successful. The appeal of St. John's wort is that the cost of trying it may be small compared to the cost of trying a prescription antidepressant. One doesn't need a prescription, and therefore a doctor's visit, to acquire it; it has few side effects, whereas some of the other antidepressants have many; and it doesn't come with the stigma that many people associate with the need to take psychiatric medications. It's easy to give St. John's wort a try, and if it makes us feel better, we may not be so concerned about gaining a full understanding of why—or what was "wrong" with us in the first place. If a friend says, "It cured me of the blues," it's understandable that we might give it a shot if we too would like to feel a little less melancholy. "It can't hurt," we believe. Generally that is a valid assumption. But as we explain on pages 37, 39–40, and 86–87, it can be dangerous to sweep more serious symptoms under the rug by self-prescribing over-the-counter herbal remedies, and there have been some reports of more serious side effects, such as mania.

Can St. John's Wort Cure Depression?

That is certainly the hope of people like Cliff. Taking even a presumably safe, over-the-counter medication indefinitely might seem a disturbing prospect. But no medicine will "cure" depression in the same way that an antibiotic cures us of illness ridding our bodies of infecting bacteria. Antidepressants work more like medications that control high blood pressure: they suppress the symptoms and perhaps prevent further complications from an untreated illness, but if stopped too early, their absence might cause a relapse. Some recent work by Dr. Gordon Parker, an Australian psychiatrist, suggests that antidepressant drugs mobilize a recovery process that follows a typical time course. Interestingly, a placebo (a sugar pill) can be helpful in as many as 30 or 40 percent of depression cases, perhaps because an individual who finally makes a decision to do something about his or her problem by consulting a doctor begins to mobilize hope, and thereby ends the downward depression spiral.

Wendy, a 57-year-old married lawyer who originally sought treatment because of worry, tension, and frequent low mood, illustrates typical ways that antidepressants might be used to treat depression. When she was depressed, Wendy's interest in life would plummet. She found it difficult to pursue her painting, which under normal circumstances is something she enjoyed greatly, or to get interested in sex. She found herself procrastinating because of lack of initiative and keeping a very messy home. Her sleep was also disturbed. Wendy had tried a number of treatments, including the tricyclic antidepressant drug Surmontyl (trimipramine) at a dose of 75 mg, Buspar (buspirone) at up to 90 mg per day, Serzone (nefazodone) at up to 100 mg per day, and Neurontin (gabapentin), an anticonvulsant drug sometimes used as a mood stablizer, at 800 mg per day. Some of the medicines had produced unacceptable side effects, including memory impairment and fatigue, and so had been discontinued. A course of treatment with the natural remedy kava had not helped Wendy. She also mentioned in passing that the herbal treatment feverfew (used for migraine prevention) had not been helpful for her occasional headaches. Wendy was therefore somewhat skeptical that another natural remedy could help her. At our urging, she did finally agree to take 900 mg per day of St. John's wort. This dosage provided some slight benefit. Increasing the dose to 1,800 mg per day produced a substantial improvement, increasing Wendy's interest, energy, and enjoyment of sex. She also became less irritable and snappish. For Wendy, St. John's wort proved to be a remarkably effective treatment that had no negative side effects.

Wendy continues to take St. John's wort—she has now been taking it for more than a year—because both our own clinical experience and others' research have shown that a fairly long course of treatment is the best protection against relapse. About two-thirds of those diagnosed with depression recover completely from an episode, as Wendy did. The other third, who recover only partially, have a greater chance of having persistent symptoms and a greater need for longer term treatment with medications and/or therapy—perhaps for years or even decades.

Whether returning to normal functioning after one episode represents a lasting cure for you is another question. After a single episode of depression, the chance of having another one is about 50 percent. A person who has had two episodes of depression has a 70 percent chance of having a third episode. Those who have had at least three depressive episodes in the past have a 90 percent chance of experiencing a fourth episode. The time between episodes varies a great deal. There is some evidence suggesting that the periods of remission (well-being) last longer early in the course of the disorder and become shorter with increasing age. Depression is also more likely to be long-lasting, and respond less well to treatment, if some other psychiatric disorder has been present earlier, for instance, an anxiety disorder or alcohol/drug abuse.

One year after having been diagnosed with major depression, 40 percent of people still have a diagnosis of the disorder, while 20 percent continue to have some symptoms at a level below the threshold level needed for the full diagnosis. The remaining 40 percent are either symptom-free or have relatively low levels of depression.

The Scientific Evidence

How can we be sure that success stories like Wendy's are not just flukes? A 1996 *British Medical Journal* article on St. John's wort by Linde and colleagues reviewed 23 well-designed double-blind placebo-controlled trials, of which 15 compared hypericum (St. John's wort) to placebo. The hypericum used was usually standardized to 0.3 percent hypericin, the active ingredient believed to be responsible for St. John's wort's antidepressant effects. The review found that 55 percent of patients responded to the remedy whereas only 22 percent responded to placebo, a difference of over 30 percent. Typically, a placebo is likely to benefit between 25 and 45 percent of people with depression, while a drug may benefit somewhere between 50 and 75 percent. In the population studied, St. John's wort as a general rule improved the overall response in depression.

In eight of the studies reviewed by Linde and his colleagues, St. John's wort was compared to an active antidepressant (a standard form of treatment that would be used by many doctors) and performed about as well as the antidepressant. In the studies that compared hypericum to a standard antidepressant, response rates were 64 to 68 percent for hypericum and 50 to 58 percent for the standard antidepressants. All of these trials compared St. John's wort to an older style antidepressant, such as Elavil (amitriptyline), Tofranil (imipramine), or Ludiomil (maprotiline), drugs that are being used less and less in the United States today because of their side effects. In addition, a recent study by Philipp et al. (1999) demonstrated benefit for St. John's wort equal to imipramine and greater than placebo in 263 primary care patients with moderate depression.

The newer generation antidepressants, like Prozac (fluoxetine), Zoloft (sertraline), Paxil (paroxetine), and Wellbutrin, Zyban (bupropion), have fewer side effects than the older antidepressants. We do not as yet have any scientific comparisons to inform us how St. John's wort would compare with these newer drugs. It is our own clinical experience, however, that St. John's wort has even fewer side effects than the newer generation antidepressants. A large trial, funded by the National Institutes of Health and co-ordinated by Duke University Medical Center, Department of Psychiatry and Behavioral Sciences, is under way, with one of us (Dr. Davidson) serving as principal investigator. In this study, St. John's wort will be compared with one of the newer generation antidepressants (Zoloft) and placebo for eight weeks, with an extension of four months available for those who respond by the end of eight weeks. This study, which will take two to three years to complete, should provide some important answers questions about whether or not St. John's wort is comparable to newer antidepressants.

All the reports suggest that St. John's wort is close to the antidepressants in terms of effectiveness, although there are signs that its efficacy may be a little bit less. Nevertheless, we need to be cautious in interpreting these results because of several factors:

- In several of the studies, the hypericum had a distinct smell, which might have impacted efforts to keep the study double-blind, that is, to conduct it in such a way that neither the tester nor the patient knows what medicine the patient is receiving.
- These studies were very short term, which limits our knowledge of the herb's effectiveness in cases of clinical depression, where treatment is usually needed for at least several months.
- These studies were mostly conducted in patients who had mild levels of depression. While this may indicate that St. John's wort will work well for the average over-the-counter purchaser, it makes it difficult for us to compare the herb to standard antidepressants. The sample of study participants is probably quite different from that seen in most studies of depression, and the results do not tell us very much about whether St. John's wort is effective in more severe types of depression.

Why did it take us so long to discover St. John's wort if it's so effective?

There is no doubt that in the United States the love affair with St. John's wort came about only after the publication by Linde et al. of their St. John's wort meta-analysis in the *British Medical Journal* in 1996. This article brought to the attention of the English-speaking medical world the collected knowledge of the herb's use for depression in German-speaking countries. Even in Europe, however, St. John's wort was not studied scientifically until the 1970s, when a small trial was conducted in Germany to examine the effects of the herb on depressed patients and to monitor certain biochemical measures. This study showed that patients improved and that St. John's wort had measurable effects on metabolites of noradrenaline. From this study, systematic clinical trials were developed, many of them initiated by Lichtwer Pharma, a German company, which itself opened for business less than 25 years ago.

The total number of depressed patients who have taken part in clinical trials to date is fairly substantial, amounting to several hundred from the Linde analysis and subsequent studies. Typically, however, when a new antidepressant is introduced in the United States, somewhere between 300 and 1,000 subjects will have been treated in double-blind controlled trials, and as many as 1,000 or 2,000 more will have been studied in various other kinds of clinical study (e.g., open-label safety studies, long-term trials, studies of nondepressed populations, or special types of studies such as looking at the effects of the drug on heart conduction). By this measure, then, St. John's wort still lags behind the prescription drugs in terms of testing.

We still need studies to answer these questions:

- Does St. John's wort work for more severe depression?
- Is St. John's wort effective over the long term, as is often needed to treat depression?
- Which doses are best? Is 900 mg per day enough?
- With which drugs does St. John's wort have problem interactions?

Do You Need St. John's Wort?

"I'm so depressed."

We've all said this, and many people genuinely feel this way—whether they would describe themselves as "low," "gloomy," "sad," "down in the dumps," or "blue." Many of the current consumers of St. John's wort are people who recognize in themselves some of the common symptoms of depression but who do not feel disabled enough to want to see a doctor about their problem. Some such people may actually meet the criteria for one of the milder forms of depression. If, for example, you have brief spells of the blues, you may have a condition called *recurrent brief depressive disorder* (RBDD; see page 39), or something resembling it but with fewer symptoms. Some people who suffer such brief depressive spells may respond well to St. John's wort, but we really don't know very much about treating this passing psychological state. Interestingly, we sometimes find that those who experience these brief and very mild episodes of depression respond very quickly to antidepressants like St. John's wort, whereas those suffering from major depression may not notice any improvement until they've been taking the remedy for several weeks. So if you're too troubled by the blues to wait them out, you might consider trying St. John's wort.

Another common, mild form of depression is called *dysthymia*. Also described later (see page 36), dysthymia was coined from the Greek for "ill humor." It's a chronic state of unhappiness, complaining, and general pessimism that often goes on for so long that it can seem to be part of the sufferer's personality. If Kelley, the patient discussed below, reminds you of yourself, you may have this lower grade variety of depressive disorder and may benefit from St. John's wort.

Thirty-eight-year-old Kelley had felt unhappy since her teens. She could remember few sustained periods of contentment or enjoyment in life. She complained of being tired, irritable, and pessimistic. Sometimes her appetite dropped or her sleep was disturbed, but generally she had no physical problems. Kelley denied ever being suicidal but often wondered whether life had anything much to offer her. Feelings of poor self-esteem and shame were highlighted by a marriage that had arisen from a messy relationship with a man who was already married. Even before then, however, she had not felt good about herself. To make matters worse, Kelley had been laid off from her job as a loan officer with a bank because of poor market conditions. Kelley was unassertive and had much difficulty expressing her real feelings about other people, whether in a positive or a negative fashion.

Kelley began to feel much better following a one-year course of Wellbutrin (bupropion) combined with counseling, but she might have done just as well with St. John's wort. At this time, no studies of St. John's wort in dysthymia have been conducted, and we are not aware of any in the planning stage. However, since we know that regular antidepressants like Wellbutrin do help dysthymia, we would have every reason to expect that

St. John's wort might also be beneficial, because most studies that have been completed have shown it to be effective in mild forms of depression (Linde et al., 1996).

If the blues are beginning to impair your life—rendering you less able to do what you'd normally do at home and at work—you should certainly seek treatment. When its symptoms go untreated, depression takes an enormous toll in personal suffering, reduced productivity, distress to those around the depressed person, and even loss of life. A recent study by the World Health Organization placed depression as the number-one cause of disability worldwide, outstripping illnesses such as chronic obstructive lung disease (emphysema), chronic anemia, injuries, and arthritis. Affecting more than 17.6 million Americans every year, depression costs the economy over $43 billion in sick days, lost productivity, and treatment, making it as costly as heart disease.

As so many self-prescribers have discovered, it's not always necessary to put a name to your feelings of depression to benefit from St. John's wort. But just as you would not take aspirin day in and day out without questioning why you continue to have headaches, you probably should not take St. John's wort for even the mildest symptoms of depression without understanding what depression is, how it tends to behave, and when it calls for a doctor's visit. If, after about six weeks of taking St. John's wort, your symptoms haven't improved at all or enough to return you to normal functioning, see your doctor. Something else may be causing your symptoms. If you do suffer from clinical depression, you may need a different medication or a combination of medication and psychotherapy to bring you completely back to normal. And, as we mentioned earlier, even if St. John's wort seems to "cure" the blues for you, you may not have seen the last of them. Knowing what to expect can make you a smart consumer of health care products and services.

What You Need to Know about Depression

Make no mistake about it, depression is a widespread and potentially devastating disorder. Major depression is one of the most common disorders in the United States, affecting 17 percent of U.S. adults over their lifetimes, with new episodes occurring in one out of every 300 people each year. If we add up the three main forms of depression, approximately 23 to 25 percent of the U.S. population will have experienced at least one of these disorders at some point in their life. Depression has apparently been with us throughout history. Michelangelo, Martin Luther, Abraham Lincoln, Winston Churchill, Emily Dickinson, Virginia Woolf, and Sylvia Plath, are just a few of the famous figures who suffered from depression, and Lord Byron is just one who was tormented by manic–depressive (or bipolar) disorder.

Major depression affects women more commonly than men. While lifetime rates vary from 10 to 25 percent in women and from 5 to 12 percent in men, the rates of major depression in the population at any one point in time vary from 5 to 9 percent for women and from 2 to 3 percent for men. The prevalence of depression is not related to racial status, marital status, income, or level of education. There is evidence to indicate that the rate of depression has been increasing throughout the 20th century. (One interesting speculation as to the reason for the rise is discussed on page 60.)

Although depression eventually runs its course, or spontaneously ends, this can take a long time. The famous German psychiatrist Emil Kraepelin observed an average depression length of one year in his depressed patients more than 70 years ago. As we get older, our depressions last longer—which may explain why modern Americans, dominated as we are by an aging baby-boom generation, are so interested in finding a reliable, benign treatment for depression's symptoms.

Clinical depression has been described as "the black dog," "the dark night of the soul," "running on empty," and, in a recent book by William Styron, as "Darkness Visible." Clinical depression, or depressive disorder, is distinguished from normal sadness in that it lasts longer than could reasonably be explained by the original trigger. For example, a child may understandably become "depressed" following the death of a beloved pet. But when the sadness and other symptoms persist six months or a year later, we have good reason to suspect that the child is suffering from a mental disorder rather than the normal grieving process.

Depression can be triggered by anything, from physical illness or change (e.g., a stroke) or an underlying medical condition such as hyperthyroidism, to a traumatic event or a stressor such as divorce or the loss of a loved one. Even a pattern of negative thoughts might lead to depression. But whether the depression triggered by one of these events lasts or recurs may depend on how predisposed you are to depression in the first place (see box on page 34).

Are You Predisposed to Depression?

Genetic Vulnerability

Many people with depression can identify somebody in their family who also had the same disorder. If one member of an identical twinship has major depression, there is a 50 to 90 percent chance that the other twin will eventually develop the same illness. Since identical twins share the same genetic makeup, we conclude that there can be a genetic predisposition to the illness. In a person with depression, the rate of depression in first-degree relatives (i.e., parents, siblings, or children) can be over 30 percent.

Personality Factors

Eysenck and Metcalfe, two British psychologists, have studied some of the ways in which a depressed person may differ from nondepressed others in personality. Eysenck had coined the term *neuroticism* to describe a person who is easily upset by stress, is guilty and self-blaming, has a tendency to experience more distressing feelings than others, and generally has a "thin skin." Those who suffer from depression often display higher levels of neuroticism than other members of the population, and these levels increase even more during the depression.

Traumatic Early Experiences

Children who experience psychological or physical abuse from their parents and lack of affection may also be at greater risk for developing depression in later life.

I have friends who've taken Prozac to get them through a tough period following a traumatic loss. Would St. John's wort help me the same way?

This is a tough question to answer, because doctors differ strongly in their philosophies about prescribing antidepressants to help patients get through difficult life experiences. Some believe that treatment with an antidepressant drug, such as Prozac, can prevent people from becoming debilitated by grief; others feel that psychiatric drugs will just muffle a patient's emotions and thereby stall the grieving process, which will have to be completed eventually. We believe that severe grief, which impairs function, calls for vigorous treatment and that an antidepressant is often appropriate. St. John's wort could be useful here, although so far we do not have strong scientific evidence in favor of either St. John's wort or conventional antidepressants.

My father recently had a heart attack. He is now very depressed, despite the fact that his prognosis is very good. His doctor said he could prescribe an antidepressant, but I'm worried about adding more side effects to those his other medications might already cause. Should I suggest St. John's wort instead?

Severe depression should be treated whether or not it has been "provoked" by a particular event. In fact, after a heart attack, the treatment of depression is most important as a factor in overall recovery, since the diagnosis of depression is one factor predictive of mortality in heart disease. The challenge is to find and use the safest possible effective treatment. Some antidepressants, such as the old tricyclics, are capable of interfering with normal heartbeat, but newer drugs, such as the SSRIs and Wellbutrin, are considered safer. In a study of high-dose (1,800-mg) St. John's wort in 209 depressed patients with healthy hearts, Czekalla and colleagues (1997) found that heart conduction was not interfered with, whereas the control drug, Tofranil, produced changes that would be of concern in heart attack patients. So, Yes, possibly St. John's wort would be a reasonable choice, provided that it was effective.

My brother can't seem to stick with his 12-step program at Alcoholics Anonymous (AA), which really depresses him. We're all worried that a prescription drug would be a bad idea for a substance abuser. How about St. John's wort?

If clinical depression is present, St. John's wort could be helpful. In Chris's case, it made a positive difference. Chris had been depressed on and off for years. He was in a 12-step AA program and was leery about taking prescription medicine. He came across an article in a news magazine that mentioned that St. John's wort had been recommended for people who did not feel comfortable taking chemical medication. Chris felt so rotten that he decided to try St. John's wort, even though he had no expectation that it would help. Thus he was quite surprised when, in a matter of days, and for the first time in his life, he felt like he was going to be okay no matter what was facing him. His suicidal thoughts went away, and he found it easier to let go of situations about which he could do nothing. He felt more at ease in social settings, and became more confident.

Chris did not realize how serious his depression had been until it went away. Furthermore, now that his overall state of well-being was so much better, Chris found that he had no desire to drink alcohol. As to whether the St. John's wort impacted his alcohol cravings or just his depression, Chris did not really care: he just felt so much better!

If your brother's problem is simply one of discouragement about not being able to stick with the AA program, we do not know whether St. John's wort is likely to make a difference. One theoretical aspect, of possible interest, is that serotonergic drugs like Buspar and Zoloft have been associated with a reduced consumption of alcohol in people with anxiety disorders and alcohol abuse. So, quite possibly, St. John's wort may have a role to play too in this context, but we need to know a lot more before we can confidently recommend it in this situation.

The Various Types of Depression

There are many types of depression. Most of them are well defined for diagnostic purposes in standardized sources such as the *Diagnostic and Statistical Manual of Mental Disorders*, now in its fourth edition (published by the American Psychiatric Association, 1994). Below we provide abbreviated descriptions of these varieties of depression and discuss what we know about St. John's wort's effects on them.

Dysthymic Disorder

If you have had relatively mild symptoms of depression consistently (50 percent of all days) for two years or more, you may be among the 6 percent of the adult American population that suffers from dysthymia. As we mentioned earlier, clinicians don't yet know whether St. John's wort improves dysthymia, though it seems reasonable to guess that it would since regular antidepressants help. One of us (Dr. Davidson) took part as a clinical investigator in a large study of Zoloft, Tofranil, and placebo in dysthymic patients. In that study we found that over 50 percent of Zoloft and Tofranil subjects responded, which was significantly higher than the patients on placebo.

Bipolar Disorder

Also known as "manic–depression," bipolar disorder is a major form of depression in which the sufferer alternates between low (depression) and high (mania) periods. We would caution against using St. John's wort in bipolar disorder until more is known, since there have been reports of this herb inducing mania. If you have bipolar disorder, you should be seeing a doctor. Your doctor should prescribe a mood-stabilizing drug like lithium or Depakote (valproic acid) if you are taking St. John's wort for bipolar depression.

Adjustment Disorder

Adjustment disorder is the development of significant depressive symptoms in response to an identifiable stressor, beginning within three months after the onset of the stress and lasting no longer than six months after the stress has ended.

Again, we are short on data here, but a study by Hantsgen and Vesper (1996) found that St. John's wort was effective in patients with mild to moderate depression of no more than six weeks' duration. Although the authors indicated that their patients met the criteria for major depression, in our experience such short-duration depressions often represent adjustment disorders and can be expected to improve by themselves if one waits long enough. However, no treatment has been found to work in adjustment disorder with depressed mood, except possibly Euphytose, an herbal remedy that contains passionflower and other ingredients. So if a short-term course of St. John's wort were found to be helpful in reducing such distress, we would certainly support this application.

Does this mean that becoming very depressed after losing my husband is abnormal, and I should be taking an antidepressant?

No. Adjustment disorder is not diagnosed in the case of bereavement. Examples of stressors that would qualify for this diagnosis are the end of a romantic relationship, marital problems, divorce, parental separation or divorce, business difficulties, financial problems, losing a job, starting a new job, retirement, failure to achieve a major goal, medical illness, and bad living conditions. However, very distressing prolonged bereavement symptoms may well demand some form of treatment, perhaps even with a medication.

Premenstrual Dysphoric Disorder (PMDD)

Basically, PMDD refers to a constellation of symptoms in women characterized by markedly depressed mood, anxiety, unstable emotions, and de-
creased interest in activities. This symptom cluster must have occurred regularly during the premenstrual week (luteal phase) during the previous 12
months and must remit, or go away, within the first days of the start of
menses. While at least 75 percent of women report limited and/or isolated
premenstrual changes, about 3 to 5 percent of women are believed to experience the full features of PMDD. There is evidence that this disorder responds to regular antidepressant drugs, and we have found that St. John's
wort can also benefit PMDD.

Will St. John's wort help me if I just have garden-variety PMS?

It is reasonable to expect that treatments that are effective for PMDD will
be helpful for the less severe or less frequent forms of this disorder, that is,
"garden-variety" premenstrual syndrome, or PMS. Mary, a 43-year-old
woman under our care, found that doses of St. John wort up to 1,800 mg
per day substantially relieved the irritability, poor concentration, and feelings of bloat that had troubled her regularly for years in the days before her
menstrual period.

St. John's wort has helped me tremendously with PMS. Now I'm wondering if it would help my 16-year-old daughter, who also has some symptoms of PMS, though they don't seem to be as bad as mine.

Many doctors believe that response to a treatment is partly related to genetic or familial factors. Thus, if a treatment has helped you, it may help a
close relative such as your daughter. We believe, however, that a doctor
should be consulted before starting a course of self-treatment in a teenager.

Minor Depressive Disorder

Minor depressive disorder refers to one or more periods of depressive
symptoms lasting at least two weeks, but during which the patient has
fewer than the five symptoms required for the diagnosis of major depres-

sion. It is often associated with major medical threats such as stroke, diabetes, and cancer. There has been little research on the effect of antidepressant drugs or counseling in minor depression, although it makes good sense to use either, or both, of these approaches, perhaps starting first with treatments that have fewer side effects, which could certainly include St. John's wort.

Recurrent Brief Depressive Disorder (RBDD)

An episode that lasts less than two weeks but at least two days and recurs at least once a month over a year would be classified as RBDD. It has been estimated that about 7 percent of the population has experienced RBDD in the previous 12 months and that men and women are equally likely to develop the disorder, which often begins in adolescence.

Major Depression

Most people who seek out St. John's wort on their own will not be suffering from the seven symptoms of major depression. Much of what we know about antidepressants in general comes from studies of major depression, the most widely studied form of the disorder. We do not yet know whether St. John's wort is as effective as the other antidepressants in treating major depression. A study by Vorbach and colleagues that looked at St. John's wort and Tofranil (a standard tricyclic antidepressant) found that at somewhat higher doses the two treatments were equally effective. Unfortunately, since the investigators did not include a placebo in their study, it is impossible for us to say that either one of the two treatments did better than a placebo.

We are currently conducting a study at Duke University Medical Center to compare St. John's wort with Zoloft and a placebo. Our study sample includes people who have a somewhat more severe form of depression, as determined by a minimum score of 20 on a widely used rating scale for depression called the Hamilton Depression Rating Scale (HAM-D; see pages 81–82). So in this study we will be able to collect data beyond those for mild and moderate depression that we now have.

Generally, only people who suffer from milder forms of depression should be self-prescribing St. John's wort. Because of the damage that major depression can cause, you should seek the care of a doctor if you fit the following criteria:

Checklist for Major Depression

Do you have at least 5 of the 9 symptoms in Table 2? ☐

Is at least one of these symptoms depressed mood or loss of interest? ☐

Have these symptoms been present nearly every day, most of the day, ☐
for at least two weeks?

Have your symptoms caused significant distress or interfered with your ☐
work, social, family, or leisure activities?

Have other causes been excluded? ☐

Can you say that these symptoms are not due to a transient grief ☐
response following the death of someone close to you?

If the answer to all six questions is Yes, then you may have a major depressive disorder. St. John's wort could possibly play a role in your treatment, but first you should be evaluated and treated by a doctor.

Can really mild symptoms of depression grow into major depression over time?

As we explained earlier, depressive episodes seem to last longer and periods of remission seem to shrink as people get older. So by those measures we could say that depression may get worse as time goes on. Whether the mild or brief symptoms you feel now will eventually turn into major depression is less clear. Sometimes early symptoms of depression, or what are referred to as *prodromal* symptoms, develop between one and five years before onset of full depressive illness. So if you notice some of the symptoms we just described, but not all of them, or not as severely or as often, it doesn't necessarily mean you are not suffering from depression and never will. If there is a known family history, a known previous history of depression, or a clear persistence of one or two depressed symptoms for several months, you would be wise to seek professional help or to consider a short trial of St. John's wort. It also might be wise to understand whether you are predisposed to depression, according to the criteria in the box on page 40. Again, your symptoms may never worsen—in fact, they may totally disappear in time—but if you're concerned enough about them to consider trying even an over-the-counter remedy, becoming more informed may ease your mind.

Table 2. Symptoms of Major Depression

_____

Psychological symptoms

1. Feeling depressed, sad, or empty
2. Marked lowering of interest in almost all activities, also called *anhedonia*
3. Feeling worthless or unreasonably guilty
4. Difficulty concentrating or making decisions
5. Recurring thoughts of death; suicidal ideas, plans, or attempts

Physiological symptoms

6. Significant loss or gain in appetite or weight
7. Loss of sleep or excessive sleep
8. Loss of energy or fatigue

Psychomotor symptoms

9. Agitation (restlessness) or slowing down of movement or speech (retardation) visible to others

_____

I've read that depression usually begins when you're young, so what I'm feeling at 45 isn't likely to be true depression, is it?

The average age at onset is in fact the mid-twenties, but depression can begin at any age. Its causes are complex (see pages 32–34) and can take effect at any time of your life. Interestingly, the age of onset appears to be decreasing for those born more recently. We don't know why recent generations seem to be experiencing depression at an earlier age than their forebears, though we can certainly speculate that this is another consequence of higher stress levels resulting from modern lifestyle factors. Whatever the cause, *depression can occur in anyone at any time.* Always take the symptoms of possible depression seriously.

To Treat or Not to Treat?

As we mentioned earlier, depression tends to resolve itself over time in most cases. The big problem is that we do not know how long it is going to take or at what cost to the individual along the way. Beyond the age of 50, the average length of a depressive illness is three years, and this average length tends to increase as we get older. Significant damage can be done during these prolonged episodes. So, in deciding whether you need treatment, your most important task is to determine the severity of your depression.

How Bad Do You Feel?

Mild Depression. If you have mild depression, you won't be disabled. You may still find yourself remaining fairly productive at work, not losing time, enjoying some things but not others, and going about your daily life with respect to your family and friends. You may, however, be aware that you are functioning at or feeling only 70 or 80 percent, even if this is not apparent to others.

Moderate Depression. A more moderate level of depression occurs when you find it more difficult to get things done, procrastinate, have trouble getting started, or are perhaps losing more time from work or failing to accomplish things that might normally be expected as part of your job. Reduction in personal and social activities, withdrawal from family activities, and cessation of things like going to church and attending social functions would all be signs of a more moderate level of depression. You may not want to engage in conversation with others in the normal way. When your depression is this severe, normally your family, close friends, or colleagues will have noticed some changes.

Severe Depression. More severe depression will result in more serious impairment both at work and socially. The individual may contemplate suicide, perhaps even make plans to end his or her life. Some severe depressions can result in such a marked loss of appetite that a person's nutritional status can be in jeopardy, especially if the individual is older, for the elderly can easily become dehydrated. At this level of severity, depression can become a serious medical emergency for which treatment should not be delayed. Indeed, it may require hospitalization.

Severe depression should always be treated by a doctor. Mild or moderate depression may benefit from a doctor's advice or from self-treatment with St. John's wort.

John, a 40-year-old business executive had been feeling under the weather for about four months. He felt blue at times, describing these periods as happening about every three or four days and lasting one or two days. During these "blue" periods, he would have little to say to his wife and children, and he would not want to join his fellow executives at lunch or coffee breaks. Then he would brighten up for a few days and be his normal self. On his "down days," he would also have difficulty sleeping and consequently felt tired all the time. John believed his symptoms were related to difficulties he was going through with his father, who had recently been recently paralyzed by a stroke. After he spoke to a friend about his condition, John decided to take St. John's wort at a daily dose of 900 mg. After taking it for two weeks he felt better; after taking it for two months he found that he had not experienced any blue days or sleepless nights. He now felt back to his old self and worried less about things over which he had no control.

Warning Signs That Depression Needs Prompt Treatment

- Suicide thoughts, plans, or attempts
- No appetite, marked loss of weight
- Inability to meet work or home responsibilities
- Deteriorating relationships with friends or family
- Complicating abuse of alcohol and/or drugs
- Social withdrawal or total isolation

Depression in the general population is typically mild to moderate. Yet it's important to remember that 17 percent of the population has had or will have a major depressive disorder. Currently, 2.5 percent of the population have dysthymic disorder, but we do not know how many people suffer from mild or brief forms of depression. We can, however, assume that for every person who has moderate to severe clinical depression, there will be many more who have milder forms for which they are unlikely to go to the doctor for professional help. You may very well be in this group.

Do I really need medication at all? What about psychotherapy?

Psychotherapy is certainly another option for less severe depression, whether acute or chronic. Two kinds of psychotherapy have been shown to be effective for depression: interpersonal therapy (IPT), which focuses on conflicted relationships or other current interpersonal difficulties that may be relevant to one's depression, and cognitive therapy (CT), which is aimed at eliminating depressive thoughts and attitudes. Both types of psychotherapy can be employed in conjunction with other antidepressant treatments and herbal remedies. Certainly, therapy can sometimes help in ways that the medicine or herbal treatment have not helped. If your depression is mild to moderate, you could certainly begin treatment with IPT or CT, but make sure that your doctor or therapist is qualified to treat depression.

Whether you want to start with psychotherapy, herbal treatment, or a medication is partly a function of your own preferences and philosophical beliefs as to why you are depressed or what types of treatments make the most sense. For some people, ease of access and cost factors make St. John's wort the best initial choice. We should mention, however, that regular antidepressant medication can sometimes cost less than St. John's wort, because the former is covered at a favorable rate under some health plans. If you're experiencing mild symptoms of depression—for example, you're going through an extended period of the blues, you have predictable and problematic PMS, or you're tired of having your life interrupted by brief periods of deep melancholy and low energy—you have a good reason to try St. John's wort before seeing a therapist or physician.

If I can buy St. John's wort over the counter, why would I ever choose prescription drugs?

Prescription drugs have proven effectiveness: between 60 and 75 percent of all people who take an effective antidepressant are likely to benefit substantially, and another 10 to 15 percent will show some improvement. While many of our patients treated with St. John's wort did feel better, not all of them experienced improved mood. Some people simply fail to benefit from the herb. According to the published studies from Europe, you can expect approximately a 50 to 65 percent chance that St. John's wort will be helpful to you. This percentage is a little bit lower than that associated with most of the other antidepressants. We must note, however, that the placebo response rate in the European studies was also somewhat lower, and that the actual difference between St. John's wort and placebo, approximately 30 percent, compares favorably with the differences between the placebo response rate and the antidepressant response rate in studies of conventional drugs.

Since St. John's wort alleviates symptoms of depression for many people, it makes sense for you to take advantage of its ready accessibility and relatively low cost. The key is to be able to recognize the signs that your depression is more severe, that other problems may be at work, or that St. John's wort is not working for you. That's why we have listed all the warning signs of major depression, described the various forms of depression, and given some background on what predisposes people to depression and what its typical course is. We offer information about judging whether the remedy is working for you on pages 32 and 42. If you're going to self-treat a condition that can be serious, you need to be able to tell when you need more help.

Many people chose not to treat their symptoms of depression at all until St. John's wort became widely available. Some of these individuals had a strong philosophical preference for herbal remedies—because they grew up with folk medicine, or they had adopted a holistic lifestyle, or they had had a negative experience with traditional Western medicine—and refused to take any prescription drug that they considered less than essential. Others did not view themselves as ill but were drawn to St. John's wort by testimonials that promised greater energy, more enthusiasm, and greater enjoyment of and success in life. In both cases, if these people are getting the benefit they desire, without suffering troublesome side effects, they certainly don't need to consider prescription drugs as an alternative. Prescription drugs can have many side effects, as we'll discuss on pages 66–67, so for some people they may be preferable only if St. John's wort does not work.

If St. John's wort is improving my friend's life, shouldn't it help me too?

That depends on how similar your problems are. But even if you share the same symptoms of depression, with the same severity, the effectiveness of any treatment will vary from one person to the next. If the person who has recommended St. John's wort to you is a close relative, however, you may stand a better chance of getting the same benefits. As we noted earlier, there is some evidence that if you have a relative with depression who has responded positively to a particular type of drug, you too may be helped by the same treatment. We're not sure why—there may be genetic factors related to how your body responds to drugs, or a positive expectation may influence your response, in something similar to a placebo effect.

Who Should **Not** Take St. John's Wort?

Do not take St. John's wort if:

- *You are pregnant, trying to become pregnant, or breast feeding.* There is a possibility (based on one study in rats only) that it stimulates contractile activity in the uterus. Moreover, the effects of St. John's wort on the fetus when a pregnant woman takes the herb have not been studied.
- *You are taking therapeutic ultraviolet light treatment.* St. John's wort sensitizes the skin and makes you more susceptible to sunburn.
- *You are taking MAOI antidepressants like Nardil or Parnate* (see page 25).
- As with any drug, discontinue use of St. John's wort if you're not getting any benefit from it. (See pages 77–80 for ways to judge whether you're improving.)

Can St. John's wort do anything for me even if I'm not depressed?

This is an intriguing question. Undoubtedly, many thousands of people are self-medicating with St. John's wort to feel better, to cope more effectively with stress, or to generally improve the quality of their lives. The available research studies were conducted mostly on people under a doctor's care who had been diagnosed with mild to moderate depression. We are unaware of any studies that have looked at relatively healthy people who are aiming to improve the quality of their life or to cope more effectively with stress by means of St. John's wort. Although a study of this type has been conducted with kava (see Chapter 2), such work has not yet been conducted with St. John's wort.

Given that St. John's wort is not expensive, and that it has few side effects, it certainly may be worth a trial in this type of situation. It may possibly help healthy people to feel even better and to function more effectively; this remains a testable and important question. If you are seriously thinking of taking St. John's wort for this purpose, then it would seem reasonable to try a dose of 900 to 1,800 mg per day for a period of perhaps of two to three months. If it has failed to help you by the end of this time, you can assure yourself that you have given it a reasonable try.

Can St. John's wort help me lower stress?

Aspirin is a wonderful medicine. It will alleviate your headache, reduce your temperature, and relieve troublesome aches and pains. On the other hand, if you do not suffer from headache, high temperature, or pain and you nonetheless take aspirin, you will not notice any of these positive effects, and you may even notice some negative ones. But, on a more subtle level, aspirin might still be doing you some good, in that it serves as a blood thinner and may be helpful in reducing the risk of blood clots. Many doctors recommend taking a small dose of aspirin daily, specifically to reduce this risk. Could something similar be true for St. John's wort? If you are not depressed, taking St. John's wort will not make you any more cheerful or happy, but can it at some level help enhance your body's ability to cope with stress? The answer to this fascinating question remains unknown. Studies need to be done to establish whether or not this in fact happens.

Many people do believe that taking St. John's wort helps them to cope better with everyday stress. Since it is generally an inexpensive remedy, and its side effects are minimal, we are not particularly critical of this practice. We definitely want to put in a plea for sponsors and researchers to get together and do the necessary trials. Stress management by means of behavioral techniques is often effective. Since there are not many conditions that respond well to behavioral therapy, yet remain unresponsive to medications, the logic for pursuing such trials is strong. In other words, most conditions that respond to behavioral forms of treatment also respond to certain medications. For more on stress management using herbs, see Chapter 2.

I have a short fuse and lose my temper a lot. Would St. John's wort help?

Irritability, anger, loss of temper, and (in some cases) even violence may be manifestations of depression. Psychiatrists in the 1960s grouped depression into anxious, retarded (i.e., slowed-down), and hostile types. Our own work at Duke University has produced similar findings. The emotion of irritability has been neglected in descriptions of depression and does not even feature in the diagnostic criteria. But this is not to say it is not important; on the contrary, it can be an important symptom and definitely one that is very disruptive and disturbing to family members and friends of the affected person.

St. John's wort probably would help if the anger were part of a depression. It might also help for other people whose anger is based on some other mechanism, such as anxiety, given that St. John's wort has serotonin-modulating effects (for more discussion of this neurochemical effect, see page 59). However, more work is needed to settle this question. Meanwhile, if you have problems with irritability or a short temper and you wish to try St. John's wort, we would suggest that you monitor its effect by means of the Visual Analogue Scale shown on pages 79–80. If it has failed to help after several weeks, then you may want to consider a medical consultation.

More Than an Antidepressant . . . But How Much More?

We've now seen that there are many forms of depression and that depressive symptoms are wide ranging, from eating problems to sleep problems, from anxiety to exhaustion, from low self-esteem to low optimism, from sadness to irritability, and much more. St. John's wort can apparently help with all of these symptoms, though we do not yet know whether the herb is more effective for some forms of depression than others. However, from our knowledge of the effects of St. John's wort on various brain chemicals (see Table 1 and pages 57–61), we might theoretically expect that it would be helpful not only for pure depression but also for depression accompanied by panic attacks, avoidance of crowds or public places, and avoidance of being the center of attention.

We also have evidence of other positive uses for the herb. It is not uncommon for a medicine brought out for one particular problem to be found useful in a wide range of other disorders. St. John's wort is no exception. There is evidence, for example, that it can be helpful in insomnia, seasonal affective disorder, and anxiety.

St. John's Wort for Sleep

While no formal studies have been conducted, Cass (1997) has reported on the benefit of St. John's wort in promoting good-quality sleep. St. John's wort can be helpful for the treatment of mild insomnia in the absence of depression—this is an interesting effect considering that some prescription antidepressants actually *cause* insomnia. It carries some advantages over many traditional sleep-promoting drugs: it does not produce morning hangover or daytime drowsiness, nor does it produce physical dependence. No withdrawal symptoms have been reported after stopping St. John's wort.

St. John's Wort for Seasonal Affective Disorder

Seasonal affective disorder (SAD) is a term used to describe people who are prone to developing depression during the winter months. SAD has been well described in Norman Rosenthal's *Winter Blues*, which describes, among other things, the benefits of light therapy for this condition. In a study by Kasper and colleagues (1997), 900 mg of St. John's wort was associated with significant lowering of the HAM-D score (see page 49); the addition of bright light therapy (a more conventional treatment for SAD) did not add any further improvement, suggesting that hypericum, the active ingredient in St. John's wort, was an effective and also well-tolerated treatment for this disorder. The same investigators had done a similar study with Prozac, in which they found Prozac to be largely equivalent to hypericum. It is a very reasonable approach, then, to treat SAD with brief courses of St. John's wort treatment.

St. John's Wort for Anxiety

Unfortunately, no good scientific studies have addressed the use of St. John's wort for treating anxiety. However, in our own clinic, we have used St. John's wort successfully as a treatment for people with anxiety disorder. It does appear to have anti-worry effects and to promote better management of stressful situations. Also, a number of people with obsessive–compulsive disorder have told us that St. John's wort has helped them, particularly with their mood in coping with the disorder.

St. John's wort might help with anxiety for several reasons. First, almost all antidepressants are effective for treating anxiety, even in the absence of depression. Second, the flavonoid component of St. John's wort has been identified as producing anti-anxiety effects. Third, we now know that hyperforin may be an important antidepressant element in the plant (see pages 55–57); indeed, it would be interesting to examine whether hyperforin alone accounts for the plant's anti-anxiety effects.

Many primary-care doctors in family practice see patients with mixed states of depression and anxiety. St. John's wort may help with this disorder since it affects two chemicals known to be involved with anxiety and depression: noradrenaline and serotonin. Unfortunately, treatment studies of mixed anxiety–depressive disorder are few and far between, so we have no real data to inform us about the best treatment. While researchers are looking more deeply into St. John's wort for the treatment of sleep disorders, SAD, and anxiety, they are also beginning to consider some of the many historical medicinal uses of the herb.

Did Our Forebears Know Something We Don't Know?

St. John's wort, or *Hypericum perforatum*, has been a folk-medicine staple for thousands of years. Its bright yellow flowers blossom around Midsummer's Day, perhaps suggesting magical properties to our ancestors. Ancient herbalists may have thought that the plant contained some of the life-giving forces of light.

The mood-enhancing effects of this plant have been known for over 2,000 years. Hippocrates, Pliny, Galen, and other classical writers described its other medicinal properties, including its wound-healing, diuretic, and pain-relieving effects. St. John's wort is said to take its name from the knights of St. John of Jerusalem, who took medicinal preparations of the plant on their crusades, using it to treat wounds from battle. The plant's leaves contain glands that look like tiny punctures when held up to the light; these puncture marks gave rise to the "perforatum" part of the name. The puncture marks could be described as "wounds," and may through belief in sympathetic magic have been assumed to be helpful in treating wounds. In fact, even today, St. John's wort is used by homeopathic doctors for this purpose.

So far the only conclusive research done in this country has focused on St. John's wort's antidepressant properties, but our forebears had the right idea when they recognized the herb as having multiple therapeutic properties. St. John's wort has been seen to reduce the craving for alcohol. It has been said that St. John's wort provides relief from pains, muscle cramps, premenstrual symptoms, and tissue damage caused by injury. St. John's wort has been used to help soothe damaged skin from inflammation and burns. One promising use of St. John's wort is in HIV/AIDS conditions. A number of tests have been done in this area, but the jury is still out. St. John's wort has a potential antiviral role. The prescription antidepressants, as far as we know, cannot make the same wide-ranging claims. Let's look more closely at what we know about historical claims for St. John's wort.

Can St. John's Wort Help Bacterial and Viral Infections?

The xanthones and floroglucinol components of St. John's wort have anti-bacterial properties. Perhaps this explains why St. John's wort has been found to be as potent as the sulfonamide antibiotics. However, at this time, with the absence of adequate scientific proof, we would not recommend St. John's wort for the treatment of bacterial infections.

With respect to viral infections, there is some evidence that hypericin has effects against retroviruses, such as the herpes simplex viruses I and II, which cause cold sores and genital herpes, respectively. In an ongoing study at New York University, Dr. Daniel Meruelo and his colleagues are evaluating whether or St. John's wort might be helpful for combating the human immunodeficiency virus (HIV) infection, as well as AIDS. Studies in animals have shown that hypericin can inactivate the virus and even protect healthy cells from attack by the HIV virus. In one small study of blood contaminated with the HIV virus, the application of hypericin led to inactivation of all the contaminating virus.

Regarding studies of AIDS patients, one found that the use of St. John's wort led to a modest increase in the number of T cells, a critical fighting element of the immune system (Cooper and James, 1990). In another study, CD-4 cells, another component of our body's natural defenses, improved after AIDS patients' prolonged use of St. John's wort (Stenbeck-Klose and Wernet, 1990). Of the 16 patients on this herbal remedy, only two developed opportunistic infections that complicated the course of AIDS. We should note that these studies were done with synthetic hypericin and not the whole herb. (The use of intravenous synthetic hypericin for AIDS studies produced troublesome sunburn, which limited the dose and therefore the effectiveness of this treatment in AIDS.)

Does this mean taking St. John's wort might actually protect me from getting colds and flus?

We do not have any evidence that taking St. John's wort will protect you from getting colds and flus, but it is an intriguing idea!

Does St. John's Wort Help Wound Healing?

The anti-inflammatory effects of St. John's wort may be due to the flavonoids. The German Commission E monograph suggests use of St.

John's wort for the treatment of injuries and first-degree burns (those that affect the top layers of the skin). In this case the remedy is applied externally, in topical form, as an ointment or oil. St. John's wort may even reduce blood loss following surgical operations.

The ability of St. John's wort to heal wounds is one of its oldest reported effects. First-degree burns have recently been found to heal more rapidly when treated with a St. John's wort ointment. More severe burns, when treated with a St. John's wort ointment, did not develop troublesome scar tissue, which sometimes complicates burn healing. St. John's wort also compares well against calendula, a widely used herb for wound healing.

Bruises and sprains have also been found to respond to St. John's wort, which seems to promote healing in this regard, perhaps due to its anti-inflammatory effects (i.e., its ability to reduce swelling, heat, redness, and pain). It may also help to heal bruising because it strengthens blood vessels and helps to repair damaged vessels.

Is St. John's wort ointment easy to find? My stores seem to have dozens of brands of tablets and capsules, but I haven't seen any ointment.

Ointments, used mainly for wounds, injuries, and postmenopausal complaints, do exist. If you can't find any in your stores, consider contacting a manufacturer directly.

Looking Ahead

We can look into the future with hope that we will be able to demonstrate convincingly that St. John's wort has many uses that we haven't even discovered yet. Its flavonoids suggest that it may have anti-inflammatory, diuretic, tumor-inhibiting, and blood-vessel-strengthening properties. Its hypericin and pseudohypericin may have antiviral properties and therefore be useful in conditions such as AIDS, hepatitis, herpes simplex virus, and Epstein–Barr virus (which causes chronic fatigue syndrome). Its xanthones may reveal that St. John's wort could become a useful, and perhaps safer, more "natural" antibiotic, as would also be the case for the fluoroglucinol derivatives. The burn-healing effects of St. John's wort may be explained by the carotenoids present in the compound.

I've heard so many claims for what St. John's wort can do. What should I expect it not to do for me?

St. John's wort probably would not be a helpful treatment for people suffering from hallucinations or delusional ideas, for example, ideas of persecution or the belief that one's mind is being controlled by external agents, as is sometimes seen in schizophrenia and related disorders. St. John's wort would not be useful for anyone suffering from mania or hypomania. This raises the question of whether St. John's wort would in fact be an appropriate treatment for the depression associated with bipolar disorder. It is known that many antidepressants can trigger episodes of mania in such individuals. The same might well be true of St. John's wort. There have certainly been some case reports. A 75-year-old widower with a history of bipolar disorder whom we had seen had been treated successfully with lithium and Prozac. He decided to discontinue his Prozac himself and then put himself on St. John's wort. Shortly afterward he started to experience more episodes of mania, and several months passed before he got back into medical care. His doctor discontinued the St. John's wort, thereby bringing his manic episodes under better control again.

There are a wide range of conditions for which the use of St. John's wort has not been studied. Therefore claims for its efficacy cannot be firmly made. However, for many of these conditions, there is some indirect evidence that St. John's wort may indeed be helpful. These conditions include anxiety disorders, premenstrual dysphoric disorder, and SAD—all discussed earlier.

Can I use St. John's wort to lose weight?

Some people have claimed that St. John's wort is useful in combination with ephedra (or ma huang) as a kind of natural weight-reducing formula. We caution against combining St. John's wort with ephedra, because ephedra has been associated with serious toxicity, including irregular heartbeat and increases in blood pressure, and with psychosis, including hallucinations and persecution delusions. St. John's wort is sometimes included, along with ephedra, in herbal weight-reducing products. In fact, the FDA has issued warnings about its use for these reasons. Regarding St. John's wort alone, we know of no evidence that it contributes to weight loss. St. John's wort is probably mistakenly associated with weight reduction because antidepressants can at times reduce overeating in those people who have a clinical depression in which overeating and weight gain are symptoms.

Can children take St. John's wort?

St. John's wort has not been studied in children. All studies have been conducted in adults, primarily between the ages of 18 and 65. Of course, regular antidepressants have been studied with children, and proven to work well. We do not, however, recommend that you treat your child with St. John's wort on your own. Discuss the idea with your child's doctor first, and explore all the possible options before you make a final decision. We agree with Thase and Laredo (1998), who have stated that with children it is important to give due consideration to all legitimate and effective forms of treatment, including counseling, therapy, and regular antidepressant drugs, as well as St. John's wort. If your child's doctor and you decide to move ahead with St. John's wort, you will have to pay close attention to both progress and tolerance of the remedy.

Thase and Laredo suggest that for a child below the age of 10 half the adult dose is a reasonable starting point, and that from the age of 15 on the full adult dose is reasonable. Between ages 11 and 15, somewhere between three-fifths and four-fifths of the full adult dose would be recommended.

While St. John's wort probably does not have as many side effects as prescription antidepressants (see pages 66–67), this has not been proven in children. You must remember that, as an active medicine, St. John's wort certainly has the potential to cause some side effects, as well as to mix with other medicines.

Can older adults take St. John's wort?

Regarding patients above age 65, it would be wise "to start low and go slow" with the dose. In many cases, it will be possible to eventually reach the full dose of 900 to 1,800 mg per day. Again, there is no real scientific evidence to guide us about the maximum effective safe dose for people in this age group.

As we age our livers become less able to metabolize drugs and our kidneys become less able to remove these breakdown products from the body. This means that older individuals are more at risk than younger ones for developing medication side effects.

Other points to consider for older people are that (1) depression may be more likely to reflect some other underlying medical problem (e.g., low thyroid activity or other hormonal imbalance, dementia, vitamin B_{12} deficiency or other metabolic problems, or cancer) or psychiatric disorder; (2) other medical problems may already be present, making it especially important to have a medical consultation; (3) medication may be causing depression as a side effect or as an interaction; and (4) suicide is a particular risk of depression in older age groups.

✒ HOW ST. JOHN'S WORT WORKS

St. John's wort (*Hypericum perforatum*) is one of more than 300 species in the hypericum family. So far only this one species has been demonstrated to benefit depressed people. A perennial herb, it grows in woods, fields, and hedgerows, particularly in lime-rich soil, the world over. It is known as *Sint Jan's kraut*, in Holland, as *herba de millepertuis* in France, as *perforata iperico* in Italy, and as *quian ceng lou* in China. Exactly what is in St. John's wort? What accounts for its many medicinal properties?

The bright yellow flowers of St. John's wort are composed of chemical substances that are potent medicines that may be helpful for several disorders besides depression. These components are all listed in Table 3, which reveals how this remarkable plant can help to relieve infections, anxiety, and depression and to open up narrowed blood vessels.

You'll notice that other substances in the plant are listed in the table as antidepressants. It wasn't always so. For a long time scientists believed that hypericin was mainly responsible for the plant's antidepressant properties. That's why the St. John's wort available on the shelves today has been

Table 3. St. John's Wort Components and Their Actions

Components in the plant	Suggested action
Hypericin, pseudohypericin	Antidepressant
Hyperforin	Antidepressant
Flavonoids	Anti-anxiety, antiviral, blood vessel strengthening
Promethocyanidins	Antibacterial, vasodilatory
Fluoroglucinols	Antidepressant, antibacterial
Xanthones	Antiviral
Carotenoids	Burn healing

standardized for its hypericin content—as most labels state. A recent study of St. John's wort by Chatterjee et al. (1998), however, suggests that another compound, hyperforin, may also contribute to its antidepressant effect. Hyperforin comprises about 4.4 percent of the ripe fruit and 2 percent of the flower of St. John's wort. In one study, a preparation containing 5 percent hyperforin was associated with a positive response in 49 percent of patients; a preparation containing 0.5 percent produced a 39 percent response rate; and placebo produced a 33 percent response rate. Side effects were few. In the 5 percent hyperforin group ($N = 49$), rates of side effects were 29 percent in the hyperforin group and 31 percent in the placebo group.

So one study that looked at hyperforin has concluded that it is the substance primarily responsible for the antidepressant effects of St. John's wort. While the study was well designed and carefully carried out, it was only one study. At the present time, the most truthful thing to say is that we do not yet know which of the many ingredients in St. John's wort is responsible for the plant's antidepressant's properties, but that hyperforin looks like a promising candidate. This means we know that hypericin-standardized St. John's wort is an antidepressant, but that the plant's antidepressant property may stem from whatever hyperforin is in the product, not from the hypericin. Of course, even if hyperforin is most responsible for the antidepressant effects of St. John's wort, we do not know whether it might also explain some of the other benefits, such as its effects in anxiety and premenstrual dysphoria.

For the purposes of understanding how St. John's wort works, we need to be aware of an elaborate chain of events that lies between the growing leaf and the capsule in the bottle. Some events are influenced by variables we have very little power to control, such as the weather, and others we can influence to a greater degree, for example, whether the plants are planted facing north or south. In the United States, most domestic St. John's wort is harvested from the Pacific Northwest and the East, with collection usually taking place between June and September. The concentrations of hypericin and pseudohypericin are affected by handling practices, moisture levels, altitude, and the different parts of the plant. It is important to gather flowering tops soon after the flowers open because this part contains the highest concentration of the presumed active compounds. Levels of the medicinal substances also diminish rapidly after pollination has occurred. Narrow-leaf varieties of the plant provide higher concentrations of hypericin than do the broadleaf varieties.

Properly dried herbs, including flowers, buds, and upper leaves, provide the highest concentration and broadest range of relevant chemicals. If too many of the lower leaves are harvested, there is a significant lessening of active constituent. For the safety of the harvesters, and to avoid blistering on eyes and skin, it is important that they keep their hands covered and avoid touching their eyes during the harvesting process.

The fresh plant material is processed and packed under refrigeration and protected from light until it reaches its manufacturing destination. Hypericum should be dried in the shade, since exposure to direct sunlight can result in great loss of hypericin. Because *Hypericum perforatum* can be adulterated with other hypericum species, care must also be taken to prevent this from happening in the harvesting process.

Obviously, then, preparation of medicinal St. John's wort is an art form, much like the cultivation of good wine, which means that much depends on the skill of the preparer.

How St. John's Wort Acts on the Brain

St. John's wort, unlike the other antidepressants, affects five chemicals present in the brain: serotonin, noradrenaline, dopamine, gamma-aminobutyric acid (GABA), and interleukin-6 (IL-6). Serotonin, noradrenaline, and dopamine, widely present in the brain, are believed to play an important role in regulating how we feel. When we are depressed the balance of these chemicals is altered. Therefore drugs that correct the imbalance in any of these substances may be useful antidepressants. Thanks to many animal studies done on St. John's wort, we know that St. John's wort seems to fit into this group. The fact that St. John's wort affects serotonin and GABA, which are also highly involved in the regulation of fear and anxiety, may explain why St. John's wort seems to have anti-anxiety as well as antidepressant effects. IL-6, a chemical in the body's immune regulation system, is suppressed by St. John's wort. It is thought that IL-6 can regulate mood indirectly by increasing a brain hormone, corticotropin-releasing hormone (CRH). Too much CRH may be related to depression, so IL-6 suppression, which would in turn suppress CRH, may be beneficial. Interestingly, St. John's wort has a beautifully balanced combination of chemical effects, which rather than any one element may be responsible in aggregate for its antidepressant properties.

Noradrenaline

Noradrenaline is perhaps the major chemical produced in the brain in times of alarm and threat. A small area at the base of the brain, called the *locus ceruleus* (or "blue place," to give it its literal translation), serves as the body's alarm system. In any situation that requires preparation to deal with threat, or for which increased levels of alertness and arousal are needed, the locus ceruleus becomes active and releases noradrenaline. Many theorists view depression as a state of biochemical hyperarousal, which is manifested clinically with such symptoms as physical agitation and inability to sleep (or to become "dearoused" if you like). It may seem odd to describe depression as a state of hyperarousal, but in the "old days" in psychiatry people who were suffering from severe depressive stupor were in fact wide awake and experiencing what Sir Aubrey Lewis has been known to refer to as "a ceaseless roundabout of painful thoughts." Many antidepressants work by reducing activity in the locus ceruleus and slowing down the production and excretion of noradrenaline. One way this can happen is by blocking the reuptake of noradrenaline from the *synapse,* the region between two nerve cells, back into the nerve cell. St. John's wort, like some other antidepressants, works in this way. Noradrenaline has also been identified as a neurotransmitter that is very important in mediating behaviors related to social approval, affiliation, and the enjoyment of rewarding activities. As we noted earlier, however, noradrenaline is not the only neurotransmitter that is important to our understanding of depression.

Dopamine

Where noradrenaline is related to the enjoyment of rewards, dopamine is tied up with the pursuit of pleasure and pleasurable behaviors. For instance, sexual interests, cravings for pleasure-producing drugs, and some aspects of eating are thought to be closely tied to normal dopamine function. Whereas noradrenaline may be thought of as mediating the pleasures of the feast, dopamine is perhaps better thought of as having to do with pleasures of the hunt. One drug that has dopamine-regulating effects, Wellbutrin or Zyban (bupropion), has been found effective in helping people to quit or at least control their smoking. Dopamine is also intimately tied to physical activity, initiation of drive, movement, and will-related activities (volitional behavior). St. John's wort also has some dopamine reuptake inhibiting properties, which may explain part of its effects. It is also of interest that drugs that inhibit reuptake of dopamine rarely produce negative sexual side effects and sometimes can actually enhance sex drive or the sexual response.

Serotonin

Serotonin is a neurochemical that has effects related to sleep, appetite, and anger regulation, and also to anxiety and harm avoidance—all issues commonly associated with depression. Serotonin also plays an important role in sexual functioning. Serotonin regulation is faulty in many cases of depression; treatments that restore its regulation are effective. Drugs that can restore the regulation of serotonin include the selective serotonin reuptake inhibitors (SSRIs)—for example, Prozac, Paxil, and Zoloft, and other serotonin-normalizing drugs such as Serzone and Effexor. Also, the older antidepressants like tricyclic drugs (Elavil, Tofranil, and Sinequan) and the monoamine oxidase inhibitors (MAOIs; e.g., Nardil, Parnate) all have serotonin-normalizing properties; they all do several other things as well. St. John's wort is a weak SSRI, which may be one reason for its effectiveness in depression.

SSRIs and other serotonergic drugs can produce sexual difficulties such as impaired arousal and inability to achieve orgasm. Typically, 30 to 40 percent of people taking these drugs experience such negative sexual side effects, but on occasion as many as 80 to 90 percent of people may report them. The stated "official" rates are usually much lower, though, because this is one type of side effect that many people don't want to mention. Although St. John's wort is a serotonin reuptake inhibitor, actual rates of sexual difficulty associated with use of the herb are low, which may be due in part to its other workings, such as its dopamine-like effects. Drugs that restore serotonergic function also can help to promote sleep and restore appetite, as well as overcome those aspects of depression that involve fear and avoidance of any kind of risk taking. They also have anti-worry properties.

GABA

GABA, one of the most widely present neurotransmitters in the brain, is associated with inhibition of arousal and fear. It is perhaps the brain's biggest internal anti-anxiety substance. GABA is the substance activated by the widely used benzodiazepine drugs. St. John's wort, at least in animal

Depressive Foods: Can You Eat Your Way into Depression?

Associated with the changes that take place in balances of noradrenaline and serotonin (the so-called biogenic amines) in depression is something referred to as the "acute phase" (AP) response. In the acute phase response to a shock or change (such as depression), the body produces an inflammatory and immunological activation, with an increase in prostaglandins and pro-inflammatory cytokines (substances that promote an inflammatory reaction), such as interleukin-1β (IL-1β), interleukin-6 (IL-6), and tumor-necrosis factor-α (TNF-α). These three substances work together to lower concentrations of tryptophan, which is the building block of serotonin. Thus the amount of serotonin as well as the number and activity of serotonin receptors is lessened. Stressful events that give rise to depression can activate the cytokine system, which in turn effects serotonin, one of the key chemicals in depression.

What does all of this have to do with food? The prostaglandins and cytokines have to come from somewhere. They are formed from and affected by polyunsaturated fatty acids (PUFAs). PUFAs have two different kinds of effect on cytokines. PUFAs found in fish, wild game, and leaves (known as Omega 3 fatty acids) lead to a lowering of the AP response and perhaps enhance the function of serotonin. By contrast, PUFAs found in vegetable oil (known as Omega 6 fatty acids) promote the AP response, reduce high-density lipoprotein cholesterol (the "good" cholesterol), and perhaps further disturb the function of serotonin. Could diets that are rich in Omega 6 vegetable oil–derived fatty acids contribute to depression? Supporting this idea is the fact that Western diets now contain ever increasing ratios of Omega 6 to Omega 3 PUFAs, while at the same time the incidence of depression has climbed since 1913. While these are still just hypotheses, it is intriguing to think that the food we eat may directly influence our mood state and that eating more fish and green leafy vegetables may not just be "good for you" but may also be good for your depression, either as a preventive or as an adjunct in treatment.

studies, has very marked GABA-ergic effects, although it is not yet known whether these effects promote or antagonize GABA. However, it does seem quite probable that St. John's wort has a GABA-normalizing influence. This could explain how St. John's wort could be both an anti-anxiety remedy and an antidepressant, since GABA has been theorized to be important in regulating depressed mood.

Considering all the effects that St. John's wort has on the brain, do I need to worry about its interactions with alcohol or anything else?

Although there is no evidence that St. John's wort and alcohol are particularly troublesome in combination, combining alcohol with any drug that acts on the nervous system always poses a potential problem. For now, perhaps, the best advice is that moderate consumption of alcohol could be permissible with St. John's wort, just as is the case with alcohol and some other prescription medications. However, you should realize that the effects of this combination are unpredictable and be on the lookout for such things as altered alertness, impairment in performance, sedation, and disturbed sleep pattern.

You should also be careful about combining St. John's wort with recreational or illicit drugs. Cocaine and stimulants, in particular, could react with St. John's wort in unpredictable ways. The same might be said for some of the dietary preparations, like phentermine. These drugs in combination can increase the noradrenaline, dopamine, and/or serotonin in your system. Because the dose of recreational drugs is not properly controlled, there could be the risk of such things as increased blood pressure, increased agitation, and perhaps worsening of mood.

It is possible that St. John's wort may interact with prescription medicines—like digitalis, warfarin, cyclosporine (used to prevent organ rejection in transplant patients), theophylline, indinavir (a protease inhibitor used in treating AIDS), some oral contraceptives, and other as yet unknown prescription drugs—to lower the levels of these drugs and reduce their effects in your body (Ernst, 1999). Thus as we have said elsewhere, we want to remind you how important it is to let your doctor know that you are taking St. John's wort. If you are already on any of these prescription medicines, and are considering taking St. John's wort, discuss it with your doctor first.

Does St. John's wort interact with tobacco?

No studies have been done to examine this issue, so we really cannot say whether there would be an adverse effect from nicotine.

Someone just told me that if I'm taking St. John's wort I should stop eating cheese altogether. Is this true?

One of the original theories to explain the antidepressant effects of St. John's wort related to its apparent property as an MAOI. MAO, which stands for monoamine oxidase, is an enzyme responsible for breaking down (inactivating) noradrenaline and serotonin, two chemicals inside the body that are associated with mood, temperature regulation, and blood pressure control. By inhibiting MAO, levels of these substances can increase, with resulting improvement in mood state or anxiety. While MAOI are usually safe on their own, when they are combined with some other medicines or foods, such as certain cheeses, they can produce a potentially dangerous interaction resulting in high blood pressure and/or increased body temperature. Fortunately, the early studies suggesting that St. John's wort does inhibit MAO have not turned out to be clinically meaningful. In actual practice, St. John's wort is not an MAOI. As a result, there is no need to worry about limiting certain foods or carrying a long list of medicines that have to be avoided. The only medicines that we advise an absolute prohibition against are the MAOI drugs (Parnate, Nardil, Marplan), which should not be combined with treatments that have serotonin reuptake inhibiting effects.

Are there any lifestyle changes I can make that will enhance the effect of St. John's wort?

There is some evidence that a healthy diet and proper exercise can help improve depression. Exercise has been shown to help depression in a number of clinical studies. A diet higher in complex carbohydrates than in simple sugars will probably give you more energy. There is some evidence that foods rich in polyunsaturated fatty acids (PUFAs)—fish, wild game, and green vegetables—can enhance the functioning of serotonin at times of stress. But we have no evidence that any of these measures will effectively treat depression on its own or that any of them will chemically enhance the efficacy of St. John's wort.

How long will it take for all these neurochemical effects to change the way I feel?

Usually it takes between six and eight weeks to reap most of the benefits from the appropriate doses of an antidepressant, including St. John's wort, in depression. Fortunately, you will see some changes much earlier than that. For example, you may begin to worry less, feel slightly less tense, have more energy, and be more hopeful in as little time as a week. We do not know if there is any set sequence in which you can expect symptoms to improve. It is not unusual to find yourself feeling 10 to 15 percent better within two weeks, perhaps 40 to 50 percent within four weeks, and as much as 70 to 80 percent better by six to eight weeks.

More severe forms of depression take longer to improve. Relapse into a depressed state may respond more quickly, either to a dose increase or to a second drug, since the body has already become familiar with the drug from previous treatment.

Very mild states of depression, the blues, or even premenstrual syndrome can respond very quickly, sometimes within days.

How long does St. John's wort take to build up in my body? How long does it last?

In a 1994 German study by Staffeldt and colleagues, healthy volunteers were given 900 mg a day of hypericum extract for two weeks. Maximum levels of hypericin and pseudohypericin, two possible active ingredients in St. John's wort, were reached within three days. After the drug was stopped, it took about five to six days before it was all eliminated from the body.

In a 1998 study Biber and associates gave 900 mg per day of hyperforin-standardized St. John's wort to healthy volunteers for one week. Peak levels were reached by day 2, and the drug took about three days to be eliminated.

A study by Schellenberg and colleagues (1998) found that within four to eight hours of taking a 5 percent extract of hyperforin, certain brain wave changes occurred, as measured by an electroencephalogram (EEG). Increases in frequency bands known as alpha-1, beta-1, delta, and theta rhythms, two of which reflect noradrenergic (theta) and serotonergic (alpha-1) chemical activity, respectively, were observed. Remember, these are two vitally important substances as far as depression is concerned. Schellenberg et al. did not find any relationship between blood level of hyperforin and EEG activity.

Pharmacokinetic studies (those that measured drug levels in the blood and rates of drug elimination) are interesting, but they tell us only so much. First of all, they were conducted in healthy volunteers, and we can only assume that the same would hold true for depressives (a reasonable assumption, but not 100 percent certain). Second, we can fairly safely assume that after stopping St. John's wort, at a dose of 900 mg per day, it will take between three and five days to eliminate the drug, a useful clinical pointer if you or your doctor is thinking about starting something else that should not overlap with St. John's wort. Third, we do not know whether hypericin or hyperforin is most important in treating depression with St. John's wort or even if some other ingredients may be crucial. Fourth, we do not know if there is any relationship between plasma levels of hypericin and hyperforin and the antidepressant effects of St. John's wort. Finally, we know that the effects of St. John's wort on the brain can be measured within four to eight hours of a single dose, so some sort of activity gets going immediately! That presumably is good news.

If I take St. John's wort for several months, will my brain adapt to its effects, forcing me to increase the amount I take to get the same effect?

We have no evidence that it is necessary to increase the dose of St. John's wort due to any loss of effect.

Can I take St. John's wort indefinitely?

The safety of St. John's wort, and even the general tolerance of this remedy, is demonstrated mainly in short-term studies and in one longer term six-month trial. As with the case for most treatments, whether conventional or alternative, most of our knowledge is based on short-term studies. However, there is no evidence for long-term or permanent harmful effects associated with St. John's wort.

Could I ever become addicted to St. John's wort?

Fortunately, there is no evidence that you might become addicted to St. John's wort. *Addiction* refers to a behavior pattern in which a person develops a craving for a drug and will do almost anything to procure supplies of it. This does not happen with St. John's wort. Some antidepressants, however, like Paxil, Effexor, Zoloft, Nardil, and Tofranil can be followed by un-pleasant *withdrawal-like* (or "discontinuation") symptoms when they are stopped abruptly, but so far we have not heard of this happening with St. John's wort. Perhaps, now that we are paying more attention to the remedy, and both using and studying it more, we may discover that some discontinuation symptoms can occur when the drug is stopped. This can be manifested through psychological cravings and/or physiological symptoms such as a racing heart, nervousness, and sweating when the drug is unavailable or withdrawn. But withdrawal-like symptoms are not the same thing as addiction!

Is it possible to take an overdose of St. John's wort?

Yes, it is certainly possible. Until recently, because St. John's wort was not used very widely, instances of overdose were few and far between and not reported in the literature. No doubt this will change. Any drug that has the effects already described (inhibiting reuptake of serotonin, noradrenaline, and dopamine) is likely to be toxic if taken in too high a dose. We do not know, however, what threshold divides safe and dangerous levels. While we suspect that quite high doses could be taken with impunity, we really do not have a great deal of information. Drugs taken at very high doses with these effects result in disturbances of temperature regulation and heart rhythm, as well as disturbances in mental state and consciousness. It is known, however, that excessive doses of St. John's wort can produce heightened skin sensitivity to the sun and that even at therapeutic doses a degree of suntan or sunburn is achieved at 80 percent of ultraviolet light exposure in comparison to what is obtained without St. John's wort in the body. Nonetheless, it is thought that massive doses of the herb would be needed to produce a truly serious phototoxic reaction. Such phototoxicity was originally observed in animals that ingested vast amounts of the plant while grazing.

What we know less about, however, is whether toxic effects of St. John's wort may be more readily apparent when it is combined with other medications. The studies have not been done.

Side Effects

Does St. John's wort equal amitriptyline? The question of effectiveness for any medication cannot be a simple one because we cannot divorce the effectiveness of treatment from its unwanted side effects. An effective drug that has to be stopped because of patient intolerance equals failed treatment. Side effects are a fact of life for all medicines, but it is extremely rare to have to stop St. John's wort for intolerance, whereas having to do this with regular antidepressants is not uncommon. In fact, as the dose of a standard antidepressant, mainly the tricyclics, is increased, the side effects can become overwhelming and the full benefits of the drug therefore are not going to occur.

The published studies concerning St. John's wort report a few cases (less than 10 percent) of mild nausea, headache, and sleepiness. There is no evidence that St. John's wort increases the effects of alcohol, a significant advantage relative to some other antidepressants. There is also no evidence that St. John's wort has toxic effects on heart conduction, which also gives it an advantage over some of the older antidepressants. Interference with sexual functioning seems not to have been reported; this might be another possible advantage. However, unless your doctor asks carefully about sexual side effects, it is possible that you may fail to report them. Because St. John's wort inhibits the reuptake of serotonin, as does Prozac, there may be some likelihood of sexual difficulties, albeit probably a lot less than those associated with regular serotonergic drugs. Weight gain is not generally a problem with St. John's wort, nor is excessive sedation.

As with any treatment, however, the more experience we have with it, the more we learn. This means that side effects may occur that have not been recognized, Thus one needs to keep an open mind about the possibility of such side effects. For example, we have seen a case in which hair loss appeared to be related to the use of St. John's wort. As such hair loss has been noted with other psychiatric drugs, it certainly could happen with St. John's wort too.

The side effects of the prescription antidepressants, in contrast, are well documented. In fact, the tricyclic and the MAOI drugs are no longer used as first-line treatments in medicine because their effectiveness comes at too high a price in terms of sleepiness, weight gain, constipation, sexual difficulties, changes in blood pressure or heartbeat patterns, and other side effects. Side effects of the newer generation SSRIs and other drugs listed are not so severe. Consequently, more people are satisfied with the response. However, side effects certainly can be a problem. Perhaps the most common of these are difficulties with sexual function (e.g., orgasmic difficulty) or reduced sexual drive. Sometimes disruptions in sleep pattern, severe nausea, or frequency of bowel movements can also be a problem. More rarely, symptoms like sweating and nervousness can give rise to treatment discontinuation.

It is possible that you may be one of the small number of people who are exceptionally sensitive to the side effects of nearly all medications. In this case, you might have better toleration of an herbal preparation. If you are a person who has already put on a lot of weight during your depression, you may have good reason to use a drug like Wellbutrin (bupropion), which can produce weight loss in a significant number of cases. You would also want to avoid taking a drug like Remeron (mirtazapine) or a tricyclic antidepressant, which has a greater chance of causing excessive weight gain.

St. John's wort, in contrast, is remarkably well tolerated. It is associated with a very low discontinuation dropout rate due to intolerable side effects. Perhaps the most serious of all potential side effects, although fortunately a rare one, is the development of enhanced sunburn following exposure to sunlight, mainly in fair-skinned people. Studies looking at the extent to which this happens have found that approximately 25 percent less exposure to sunshine is needed to produce a level of tan/sunburn that would occur at higher amounts of sunlight in those who were not taking St. John's wort. At doses of up to 1,800 mg per day, this is not expected to be a serious or practical issue. However, if you are taking St. John's wort, you should protect your skin from too much exposure to the sun and perhaps also protect it by applying ultraviolet sun block. The occurrence of skin sensitization to sunlight as a result of St. John's wort is an interesting side effect, in view of the plant's special association with light. It seems as if both the skin and the psyche respond with greater sensitivity to light in one form or another.

In the double-blind trials that have been done to date, approximately 20 percent of patients on St. John's wort reported side effects, which is almost one-half of the 36 percent who reported side effects on standard antidepressant drugs. Dropout rates due to side effects were 4 percent in the St. John's wort group, in contrast to 7.7 percent with standard antidepressants (DeSmet and Nolen, 1996). Table 4 lists the rate of specific side effects from St. John's wort in depression.

In the *British Medical Journal* article mentioned earlier, Linde et al. (1996) found that the rate of side effects with standard antidepressants was 52.8 percent of patients, as compared to 19.8 percent in the hypericum group—a clear difference in favor of the herbal treatment. In a large study of over 3,000 patients treated in private practice, Woelk and colleagues (1994)

Table 4. Percentage Rates of Side Effects from St. John's Wort in Two Studies

	Wheatley (1997)	Vorbach et al. (1997)
Headache	7	0
Nausea	7	5
Dry mouth	5	3
Constipation	5	0
Tiredness/sleepiness	2	5
Itching	2	0
Restlessness	0	6
Dizziness	1	5

reported adverse reactions in a mere 2.4 percent, with only 1.5 percent discontinuing the herb. Gastrointestinal symptoms (0.6 percent), allergic reactions (0.5 percent), tiredness (0.4 percent), and restlessness (0.3 percent) were the most common side effects, but in all honesty these are exceptionally uncommon overall. While there is usually some variability in the reported rates of side effects for any treatment in a group of studies, one finding that simply cannot be denied is the overall low rate of reported side effects with St. John's wort. Considering that antidepressants usually are taken for long periods of time, this becomes a particularly important benefit, assuming (and this has yet to be studied) that St. John's wort can sustain its positive effects in the long run. If it can, then it has a clear edge over the prescription drugs whose side effects many people find intolerable over time.

Why should St. John's wort have fewer side effects?

We do not really know the answer but can speculate that it has a generally milder effect on the nerve cells and receptors than many conventional drugs. It does not seem to stimulate appetite to an excessive degree, it does not interfere with the conduction of the heart, and it does not have markedly sedating effects.

Will any of the side effects increase the longer I take St. John's wort?

One of the reassuring facts about antidepressants is that we have no real evidence that their long-term use causes any permanent side effects. Any difficulties that may arise due to the medicine will go away when it is stopped. Antidepressant pills and herbal remedies such as St. John's wort are not considered to be addictive, they do not cause any permanent damage to brain function, they do not destroy your ability to have feelings like sadness and joy, and they will not take away your control over things. Although we do not have much experience with long-term use of St. John's wort, there is no evidence so far of any long-term or permanent side effects.

Can I be allergic to St. John's wort?

In theory, a person can be allergic to anything. True allergic reactions to St. John's wort are rare. You would want to look for such things as skin rash, itching, shortness of breath, and tightness in the throat as signs of a true allergic reaction. Other unpleasant side effects are sometimes chalked up to "an allergic response," but these are not true allergies but mere intolerance or sensitivity to low doses of a medicine. An allergic reaction of the first type would be a sign that St. John's wort is probably not for you, whereas a pseudoallergic reaction of the second type may simply mean that more careful attention must be paid to the use of small doses. The skin reaction in sunlight can be a form of allergic response and can be dealt with by using sun block on your skin.

⚘ HOW TO USE ST. JOHN'S WORT

As we mentioned at the beginning of this chapter, it's easy to walk into a supermarket these days and walk out with some St. John's wort, but the odds are that what you purchase won't answer all your questions about how much of what form to take, when, and for how long. How will you know whether you're getting the maximum benefit from the herb or what to do if you're not? What are the differences from brand to brand? How and when do you change your dosage or stop taking St. John's wort? This part of the chapter will tell you how to use St. John's wort safely and effectively. The chapter ends with information on including St. John's wort in your treatment if you are already seeing a doctor for depression or feel you need to consult one.

St. John's Wort Preparations

St. John's wort comes in pill, tablet, and capsule forms; as a tea; as a tincture; as an oil; and as an ointment. The ointments are used primarily for su-

perficial injuries and should most definitely not be used for any other purpose than topical application. The essential oil preparations are best used
for the purpose of aromatherapy (whose practical value has not been
tested). Alcohol-based tinctures, though widely available, are a less well
studied form of treatment for depression. St. John's wort teas are less effective for depression. The best studied and most dependable forms of St.
John's wort for depression are the pill, tablet, and capsule.

Choosing among Brands

In our opinion, most herbal products can be assumed to be safe. However,
because you are trading in an industry populated by hundreds of only
slightly regulated companies, and at least a few of the companies could be
producing products of questionable quality, you would be wise to learn what
you can about the reputation and experience of the manufacturer before
deciding which brand to buy. *St. John's Wort: The Herbal Way to Feeling
Good*, by Norman Rosenthal, MD, is one useful resource. You might find it
helpful to check with your local pharmacists for additional information
about the different companies.

Most of the studies showing that St. John's wort is effective in depression have been undertaken with formulations manufactured by German
companies, including Lichtwer Pharma and Schwabe. The Lichtwer brand,
know as Kira in the United States, is the best studied. It has received inves-
tigational new drug (IND) status from the FDA, which means it has met
the rigorous standard required for use in clinical trials. While an IND
should not be confused with full approval of a new drug by the FDA for a
particular disease (the so-called NDA, or new drug approval), it does indicate that the herb has met some standards imposed by the FDA for good
manufacturing practices and good basic clinical testing for safety and pharmacological consistency.

Because dietary and herbal supplements are not regulated as closely as
FDA-approved medicines for particular diseases, brands may vary in how
much active medication they contain. Some brands may lose their therapeutic potency after several months. As we discussed on pages 55–57, we
have no real way of knowing which part of St John's wort is the active, or
"critical," part. It used to be thought that hypericin was key, which is why
the most reputable companies have standardized their brands to a certain
amount of hypericin (usually 0.3 percent, which would equal 2.7 mg in a

daily dose of 900 mg of hypericum). Now, however, some people are claiming that hyperforin is the active element. So, even if brands were consistent in terms of the total amount of whole hypericum extract they contain, as given by the milligram dose, we wouldn't be able to say with certainty that they all had the same total potency. As it is, we do know that tests have shown that some brands are much less potent than they claim to be.

Before you buy, examine the label. Make sure the label states that the preparation is a standardized extract containing a certain amount of hypericin or a certain percentage of hyperforin. This means that the manufacturer has prepared its version of St. John's wort with a specified amount of hypericin or hyperforin in each tablet. If the manufacturer is a reputable company, this should give you some assurance that from batch to batch or bottle to bottle you are getting the same amount of medication. Be leery of brands that fail to provide such information. Does the label include an expiration date? Is there a batch (lot) number? Are dosing directions given? Are they realistic? Avoid brands that give no dosing directions, as well as those that instruct you to take 300 mg once per day, which is almost certainly too low a dose, or as needed, which is definitely not the correct way to use the herb for treating depression.

What does price tell me about quality?

Brands do range in price, and even the same brand may cost different amounts depending on where you buy it. Purchasing the cheapest brand does not necessarily bring you the best bargain. Again, the most important things to look for are (1) brand reliability, (2) adequate information on the label, (3) endorsement by colleagues and friends whose opinions you respect and who are well informed, and (4) the amount of scientific data that supports the effectiveness of a particular brand.

A recent survey that we made in our own local pharmacies and health food stores provided some interesting results.

We evaluated what kind of information the consumer would be provided with if he or she went shopping for St. John's wort and wanted to compare brands. We present information on 10 different brands, obtained from three retail stores—a supermarket, a specialty grocery store, and a large discount chain—in November 1998. The six main points we have focused on are as follows: (1) dose per pill (or capsule), (2) recommended number of pills per day; (3) whether the brand was standardized to a certain level of ingredient (presumed to be an active part of the herb, although we cannot be entirely certain in some instances, e.g., St. John's wort and va-lerian); (4) whether other herbs or medicinal ingredients were listed on the label besides the principal ingredients; (5) whether the manufacturer indicated an expiration date for the product; (6) what the cost per day would be.

As Table 5 indicates there is considerable variation. We found that the recommended dose ranged from a low of 300 mg per day to a high of 900 mg per day (four brands). Others gave a range, while one indicated "as needed" and two said to take "with meals." For major depressive disorder, 900 mg per day is considered an average dose, 300 mg per day would be too little, and some people may well need 1,800 mg per day. Taking St. John's wort "as needed" is poor advice if you have major depression. We do not believe it matters whether you take it with food, unless you have side effects, which can sometimes be alleviated by eating before taking medication, which sometimes delays the rate of absorption of medicine. We do not know if the dosing directions just given are appropriate for stress or occasional mild depressive symptoms.

We were pleased to find that all except one brand were standardized for 0.3 percent or 0.2 percent of hypercin, which assures some consistency within brand. In many of the positive clinical studies, St. John's wort had been standardized for hypericin or hyperforin.

Three brands of St. John's wort contained between three and six other ingredients (such as ginseng, ginger, lobelia, vitamins, and amino acids). These additions to St. John's wort are probably unnecessary for achieving antidepressant benefit; we have no way of knowing what, if any, extra benefit or risk they confer.

Prices varied considerably. If we were to standardize the daily cost relative to a dose of 900 mg per day, brands varied from $0.27 to $2.16 per day!

We certainly recommend that, as an informed consumer, you become aware of these issues in your choice of an herbal brand. You will also want to select, as far as you can, a reliable and reputable manufacturer.

Is the expiration date important? Many of the bottles I looked at were about to expire in the near future, which made me hesitate to buy them.

Very often prescription medications remain good after the expiration date, but you can't have the same confidence in herbal treatments. Indeed, it has been suggested that many brands of St. John's wort have quite short shelf

Table 5. Comparisons of Different Brands of St. John's Wort Available in Three Different Pharmacies (November 1998)

Pharmacy	Brand	Dose/pill	Pills/day	Standardized	Other ingredients	Expiration date	Cost/day
1	A	300 mg	3 as needed	Yes	Yes (3)	No	$0.57
	B	300 mg	1–3	Yes	No	Yes	$0.20–0.60
	C	300 mg	3	Yes	No	Yes	$0.27
2	D	320 mg	3	Yes	Yes (3)	Yes	$0.33
	E	150 mg	6	No	No	Yes	$0.60
	F	300 mg	1	Yes	No	Yes	$0.20
3	G	150 mg	2–4	Yes	No	Yes	$0.13–0.26
	H	300 mg	3	Yes	No	No	$0.54
	I	450 mg	1–2 (with meals)	Yes	No	No	$0.54–1.08
	J	300 mg	1 (with meal)	Yes	Yes (6)	Yes	$0.72

lives. For that reason we recommend that you discard any St. John's wort whose expiration date has passed. It's unlikely that taking an expired pill or capsule will have catastrophic consequences, but why take the risk?

Manufacturers are competing vigorously for your dollar today, and many are offering two-for-one and similar bargains. Here's where an expiration date may matter: if you can't use up what you buy before its potency expires, you haven't gotten much of a bargain.

I've seen lots of brands of St. John's wort that combine it with another herb. Are they worth trying?

It is not advisable to take a St. John's wort brand that is mixed with many other herbal ingredients. While this is unlikely to result in any harmful side effects, the best knowledge regarding St. John's wort efficacy is based on the use of a single product. One study found efficacy for a combination of hypericum and valerian.

Is there a chance that side effects will vary among brands?

Without doing a direct head-to-head study of different brands, and giving them at the equivalent doses, we really cannot say with authority whether or not there is any difference in either rate or type of side effects. However, what can be said undoubtedly is that individual people sometimes tolerate one brand better than another. For instance, if you take St. John's wort and are troubled by headache, upset stomach, altered sleep patterns, or even skin sensitivity, you might alleviate these side effects just by switching your brand. Certainly, if you are using a combination of St. John's wort and other herbs, any side effects could be due to the other substances. One of our patients, George, had taken St. John's wort combined with lobelia and developed a nasty nausea and upset stomach, which disappeared when he went on St. John's wort alone.

How Much to Take and When

Most studies of St. John's wort have used capsules, pills, or tablets. At this time these forms seem most reliable. But those who have trouble swallowing pills can take the liquid form via a dropper. The teas have proven to be less effective for treating depression than other forms because it's difficult to determine the appropriate dose of tea. Regarding nutraceutical supplements, enriched foods and drinks usually don't contain nearly enough St. John's wort to affect depression.

Most brands of pills, capsules, or tablets recommend 900 mg per day, divided into three doses. Typical pills contain 300 mg of St. John's wort, of which about 0.9 mg is in the form of hypericin. Thus, a day's total contains 0.5 to 3 mg of hypericin. In the studies that have been done, a dose of 900 mg per day was often effective, but we don't really know if 900 mg per day is the most effective dose. Some people need as little as 600 mg per day. If you have been very sensitive to the effects of psychiatric medicines in the past, or if you suffer from panic attacks and are very sensitive in general to unpleasant physical sensations, it might be more prudent to begin at 300 mg per day and work up slowly to 900 mg per day over a period of one or two weeks.

The tincture (liquid) dose should be 2 to 4 ml three times a day. The tea should be taken in one- or two-cup amounts twice a day, which should add up to 2–4 grams of the herb.

I keep forgetting to take the pills three times a day. I often miss the midday dose, which I'd have to remember to take at work. Should I just take two at a time when I forget?

Although the manufacturers typically suggest taking St. John's wort three times a day, we have found it equally effective—and safe—when taken twice or even once a day. We do know from the pharmacokinetics of this drug that reasonable levels are still present up to 24 hours after administration, so on these grounds there really is no theoretical reason for taking it three times a day. Taking St. John's wort with meals may be a helpful reminder, especially if you're already taking any other medications with your meals. And if the problem is that you forget to pack your St. John's wort when you leave for work, try keeping an extra bottle at your workplace.

Is there a certain time of day that it's best to take St. John's wort?

No. The best route is to time your doses for your own convenience. If you are one of those rare people whose sleep is disrupted by St. John's wort, then taking it late at night would not be a good idea. If you suffer from nausea or stomach upset as a result of St. John's wort, then taking it with meals would be a good idea, since this tends to slow the absorption and thereby lessen the intensity of this symptom. Currently there is no timed-release preparation.

Is there anything I should know about taking St. John's wort that will increase its absorption or effectiveness?

We are unaware of any factors that increase or decrease the absorption or effectiveness of St. John's wort. Although some foods (such as grapefruit juice) are known to increase the blood level of some SSRIs, we do not have any evidence that St. John's wort is similarly affected.

Is It Working?

It generally takes between four and eight weeks to get the full benefit of symptom reduction with antidepressant treatments. It may take as long as four to six months to regain your full functioning at work and in social rela- tionships. But that does not mean you will see no improvement until four to eight weeks have passed. Even in the first week you may begin to feel a little more relaxed, to sleep better, to notice that your concentration and energy are picking up. Sometimes your relatives will observe changes in your facial expression, tone of voice, initiative, and optimism even before you notice them. These early observations are very encouraging and can be taken as vindicating your treatment choice. As time goes on, in your rela- tionships and work, you will notice greater improvement with socialization, conversation, and work productivity and success.

If your depression worsens during the first eight weeks that you take the herb, you should definitely see a doctor.

I've been taking St. John's wort for a month without noticing any difference. Should I give up?

Not necessarily. It's true that milder forms of depression usually respond rel- atively quickly, at least to some noticeable degree, but if you have dysthymia (see page 36), it might take eight weeks to see any real change because the longer your condition has existed, the longer it will take to im- prove. Remember, too, that you may have to wait a lot longer to see a full or significant return to normal functioning.

What should I do if I'm not satisfied with the benefits I'm getting?

Several factors could be at work if you're not getting the results you want from taking St. John's wort:

- You're not taking a high enough daily dose. To find out, if your initial dosing of 600 mg or 900 mg per day has not helped after a few weeks, you might consider increasing the dose to 1,200 or even 1,800 mg, provided no side effects have occurred. For some people the standard 900-mg daily dose is not enough, and a daily dose of up to 1,800 mg may be very effective. However, no study has compared 900- to 1,800-mg doses, so we don't have a definitive answer about the maximum effective dose. Considering that this remedy has so few side effects, doses higher than recommended on the labels can probably be taken (e.g., up to 1,800 mg/day), but we need studies to look at this problem. Higher doses should only be taken under the supervision of a qualified medical practitioner. In other words, do not self-prescribe these higher doses.
- You may not have taken St. John's wort for an adequate period of time. We know that with standard antidepressants it generally takes four to six weeks for these medications to show effectiveness. Similarly, you should expect that it may take several weeks to note demonstrable effect from St. John's wort.
- You're not taking a reliable brand. If you didn't do any research on manufacturers, do so now. If what you discover indicates that you may have made a poor brand choice, pick a new brand that meets the criteria discussed earlier and try again.
- Some other problem is at work, or your depression is more severe than you thought. You may need more than St. John's wort or a different treatment; see your doctor.

Self-Monitoring Methods

We suggest several different methods for determining whether St. John's wort is working for you. One or more may be easiest and most informative for you. One of the more common self-rating scales is that developed by our colleague psychiatrist Bernard J. Carroll, MD, which is copyrighted and can be obtained from its publisher, Multi-Health Systems Inc., by phone at 1-800-456-3003, or by email at customer_service@mhs.com.

A Medication Log

Over the first four to eight weeks, you can keep a more detailed medication log, like the one shown below. On this log you can regularly record the positive effects you feel, any negative side effects, and any changes in your mood or your response to the herb. This can be a great help, especially if you're trying to increase your dosage to get the maximum benefit and need to be able to tell when your progress has plateaued.

Medication Log

Day	Date	Dose/day	Effects
Monday	June 27	600 mg	None
Tuesday	June 28	600 mg	None
Wednesday	June 29	900 mg	Slight headache
Thursday	June 30	900 mg	Headache
Friday	July 1	900 mg	Headache went away
Saturday	July 2	900 mg	Slept soundly last night
Sunday	July 3	900 mg	Slept better

Percentage Improvement Rating

One simple question that we like to ask our patients, which is often amazingly accurate, is *How much better do you feel as a percentage compared to the start of treatment?* One hundred percent can be used as the mark for feeling as well as you can or as well as you were when you were healthy. An improvement of at least 70 percent means that treatment has done a good job. How much more you want to aim for is up to you. Many people are satisfied with a 75 to 85 percent improvement, while others are unhappy until they have reached 100 percent. Equally, sometimes, if you have had a really severe and chronic depressive state going back many years, or have known little happiness in your life, even a 50 percent improvement is regarded as very meaningful. In these circumstances, it is possible that benefit continues to occur slowly and progressively over a period of many months and that patience is the watchword.

Depressive Symptom Improvement Scale

Select only the symptoms that were troubling you before you started treatment. Check the appropriate box for each symptom to indicate how much it has improved. Leave the boxes blank for symptoms that were not present when you were depressed.

	No change	A little better	Moderately improved	Much improved
1. Feeling sad or tearful	☐	☐	☐	☐
2. Feeling hopeless about the future	☐	☐	☐	☐
3. Being low in energy	☐	☐	☐	☐
4. Sleeping poorly	☐	☐	☐	☐
5. Sleeping too much	☐	☐	☐	☐
6. Poor appetite	☐	☐	☐	☐
7. Excess appetite	☐	☐	☐	☐
8. Being critical of myself	☐	☐	☐	☐
9. Poor concentration	☐	☐	☐	☐
10. Ideas or plans about suicide	☐	☐	☐	☐

You can total the score and divide by the number of symptoms present. An average improvement score of 0 represents no change, while a score of 3 represents much improvement overall.

Visual Analogue Scale

A simple way to measure the severity of your own depression and your response to treatment is by means of visual analogue scales, analogous to taking your temperature or measuring your blood pressure. You can rate yourself on this scale before you start taking St. John's wort and on a regular basis thereafter to see how you're improving.

Here is how a few people we know described the personal experience of benefiting from St. John's wort:

Rob had started St. John's wort at the suggestion of his father, because he had experienced some fatigue, occasional sleepless nights, and lack of zest for life. A schoolteacher, he found that he did not look forward to going to work, which was unusual for him. He had seen his doctor, who pronounced him to be in good physical health, and was told correctly the he did not have clinical depression. Within about 10 days of starting St. John's wort, Rob began to notice that he could express his feelings much more easily and that

Severity Rating of Depression

Not at all depressed. I feel very well all the time.

	100
	90
	80

Depressed a little bit of the time:
Not very troublesome. I can function.

| | 70 |
| | 60 |

Quite a bit of depression, but I can function.

| | 50 |
| | 40 |

Difficult to function: Experience depression all the time.

	30
	20
	10

As bad as it can be. Everything looks completely hopeless. I don't want to live.

| | 0 |

Rating of Response to Treatment

How much better do you feel since you started taking St. John's wort?

As well as can be

	100
	90
	80

Very much better

| | 70 |
| | 60 |

Moderately improved

	50
	40
	30

A little better

| | 20 |
| | 10 |

No better

| | 0 |

the cloud that he felt hovering over him was starting to lift. He also described a change in the way he looked at things. Whereas in recent months he had seen every difficulty as an obstacle that he could not overcome, he now saw these situations as opportunities and challenges to meet.

Jenny, a 50-year-old mother of two children, had always tended to be ill-humored and grouchy, and her disposition was not related to any particular thing. She sometimes slept poorly. Her younger daughter, Susannah, had urged Jenny to do something about her "foul mood." "I've never heard an optimistic word from you," she added. Jenny started on St. John's wort and within 10 days had improved so much that, as she put it, "The difference was phenomenal. As the old saying goes, I didn't know how bad it had been until I started to get better." Jenny has found, like a lot of others who take St. John's wort for occasional or mild moodiness, that she only needs it at certain times. So Jenny takes St. John's wort for about a week at a time whenever she feels her moodiness, irritability, or insomnia bothering her. Having found she can feel so much better, she has also learned to observe and detect her mood changes much better.

Cara did not think she had serious depression but knew that she was not the person she could be. Her sleep was neither restful nor refreshing, she did not have as much energy as she would like, and she found it difficult to get motivated to do things. While she usually "went through the motions," often she would agree to do something and then back out at the last minute; her friends could not depend on her. Cara lacked self-confidence and was uncertain of herself. She would frequently procrastinate. After a friend pointed out that it was possible to have more subtle depression, Cara decided to try some St. John's wort. Cara expected, from her readings, that it would take several weeks for St. John's wort to work. She was therefore quite surprised, and very pleased, to notice within one week how much more restfully she was sleeping, how refreshed she was on awakening, and how she therefore no longer needed a midday nap. Cara said, "I have a great level of energy throughout the day. I'm no longer afraid of life. I'm motivated to do all the things I want to do. I'm who I was meant to be!"

Professional Measures

Besides the self-monitoring methods, several scales are used by professionals to measure depression. The most commonly used test for an antidepressant effect is the depression scale developed in England by Dr. Max Hamilton known as the Hamilton Depression Scale (or HAM-D). This consists of 17 questions asked by the interviewing doctor that cover a range of symptoms, including depressed mood, guilt feelings, suicidality, sleep disturbance, loss of pleasure, physical slowing down or agitation, anxiety, loss of weight, loss of appetite, loss of interest in sex, tiredness, and preoccupation with health worries. Each of these questions is rated from 0 to 2 or 0 to 4, and a total score is given.

The HAM-D is widely used in antidepressant medication studies and is supplemented by the Physician's Clinical Impressions (CGI) measure of improvement. The CGI allows the doctor essentially to decide whether or not treatment response is good enough that it would be recommended to continue, in which case the person is judged to have been a responder. Sometimes self-rating scales are used to supplement the HAM-D and the CGI, but there is no consistency in selection of any particular scale. On the HAM-D, a lessening in the score by 50 percent or more is a sign that response has been good; a final total score of 8 or less also indicates very good improvement. At the beginning of a clinical trial, a patient may typically score anywhere from 18 to 25, with scores below and above this indicating milder or more severe forms of depression respectively.

Signs of Improvement

- More energy
- Thinking positively about future plans
- Better sleep
- Brighter facial expression, more lively gait
- Calmer
- More active involvement with the environment
- Improved concentration

Is any improvement I gain likely to come gradually or in steps?

Most of the time you can expect that your improvement will come about gradually, a little bit at a time, so that after three or four weeks you can look back and see more clearly how much better you are. Improved sleep, energy, and concentration, as well as greater optimism and less frequent negative or suicidal thoughts, are generally quite easy to recognize. As you improve, you may have a few mild setbacks in which your old symptoms return or get worse. Don't worry about them unless they are persistent or severe. It may help to increase the dose at that point or, if you are under a doctor's care, to tell him or her about the setback.

This may sound funny, but I almost feel too good. Should I cut back on the dosage?

Sometimes antidepressants, including St. John's wort, can produce mania or hypomania in a person who has a diagnosis of, or who is susceptible to, bipolar disorder. Symptoms like excessive and/or inappropriate cheerfulness, rapid speech, racing thoughts, increased drive, expansive or unrealistic plans and behaviors, increased talkativeness, increased sexual activity or drive, overspending, excessive irritability, and reduced need for sleep would suggest the need to reevaluate and possibly discontinue St. John's wort. If you are not under a doctor's care, be sure to make an appointment.

I had to pack fast for a last-minute business trip and just realized I don't have my St. John's wort with me. I'll be away for a week with no way to buy more. What should I do?

If you have been taking St. John's wort for mild symptoms and not for more serious depression, it is unlikely that a week without the remedy will have major consequences. If you have been under treatment for more serious depression, it is also unlikely that major relapse will take place that quickly, but try to call your doctor to discuss the situation. If you have had previous experience with serious relapse shortly after discontinuing an antidepressant, you may need to make arrangements to obtain a supply. St. John's wort is available in practically all countries.

Remember that St. John's wort stays in your body for a few days after you stop taking it and may still provide some effect during this time.

How will I know when I've really reached the peak effect I'm going to get?

We think that there are three kinds of response you can look toward: (1) returning to your old ("normal") self; (2) feeling better than you thought possible; (3) improving, but not as much as you'd like. The first two outcomes are clear, and you will be satisfied with your treatment. The third one is trickier, because you will want to know whether you should (a) just continue on the same dose for a longer time, (b) increase the dose, (c) add a second treatment, (d) or stop St. John's wort and try something else. If, after 8 to 12 weeks of partial improvement, you still feel like you could do better, discuss it with your doctor.

I'm really strongly against taking prescription medications, and I don't really want to take the time for psychotherapy. Is there any other herbal remedy I can try for depression? What about other alternative medicine ideas?

There has been little research on other herbs for depression. Ginkgo has been found to help in resistant depressions in the elderly, but it is possible that this type of depression may be of different origin, possibly related to vascular insufficiency (impaired blood flow to areas such as the brain or heart). SAMe is another possibility, although not an herbal treatment.

Acupuncture has been studied at the University of Arizona by Dr. John Allen and his team. Preliminary findings in depression are very encouraging, and the outcome of a more definitive trial is awaited.

I feel so much better now that I've been on St. John's wort for a month. Can I stop taking it?

If you stop taking an antidepressant after only a few weeks, it is almost certain that your symptoms will return if you are suffering from major depression or chronic milder depression. If your problem is more intermittent (it comes and goes and does not last too long), such as premenstrual symptoms, winter blues, or just having a few down days every now and then, perhaps you could manage with taking St. John's wort on an occasional basis for a few weeks at the time your symptoms appear. In these circumstances, sometimes antidepressant and herbal treatments work quite quickly.

I don't want to take any medication, even an herbal, for the rest of my life. What signs should I look for that I don't need it anymore?

Few people with depression need medication for the rest of their lives, but some do. We believe that you will need medication indefinitely if you have bipolar disorder, have had more than three major depressive episodes, have had at least two serious relapses after stopping medication, or have been a chronic suicidal risk. If you are not in any of these groups and have shown a good response to your treatment, which has been sustained for at least a year, it is worth considering reducing your medication with a view to stopping. But it should be done slowly over several weeks or months. If problems develop, it is probably time to consult your physician.

When and How to Stop Taking St. John's Wort

If you are taking St. John's wort for clinical depression rather than for a milder problem like the blues, it is important to continue your antidepressant, including herbal treatment, for several months. Relapse rates range from roughly 30 to 80 percent, according to population studies, when medication is discontinued but are reduced to approximately one-half of this if you take your medicine for one year or more. In other words, continued medicine will lessen the chance of a relapse without protecting you entirely.

The more you have of the following features, the greater the chance of a relapse and also the stronger your need to remain on your treatment for a longer time:

- Partial response to treatment (while you are much better, you still have many symptoms of depression)
- Presence of other disorders (such as anxiety, eating disorder, or alcohol problems)
- Several previous episodes of depression
- Strong family history of depressive or bipolar disorder
- Very prolonged previous depression
- Poor social support
- Many current life stressors or relationship problems

Note that by *relapse* we generally mean a considerable worsening of symptoms. So even if you do not relapse, you would not necessarily remain entirely well. In other words, some symptoms could come back, and you may still find that you are feeling better if you remain on St. John's wort for a longer time. But, if your depression has not been very severe, and if you have made an excellent recovery with no symptoms, and also if your life is in good order with few stresses, there is certainly a possibility that you could stop your St. John's wort earlier than that.

*Do I need to taper off St. John's wort so I don't suffer any
withdrawal symptoms?*

St. John's wort is not addictive and does not cause any kind of physical dependence. Still, when you decide to stop St. John's wort, it is best to slowly
taper the medicine to prevent all of the symptoms from coming back too
quickly. If you slowly reduce the dose, you will have a better ability to identify and control any symptoms that might start to reappear. Although there
are no guidelines as to how long the taper should last, we would suggest
that tapering over one to two months would be sufficient. If you're starting
at 1,200 mg per day, you might try cutting down to 900 mg for the first
week or two, to 600 mg for the next week or two, and then to 300 mg for
another two weeks or so. Of course if you are taking only 600 mg per day,
you can probably taper more quickly.

Taking St. John's Wort under a Doctor's Supervision

St. John's wort's availability over the counter makes it possible for some people to self-treat effectively, at a modest price, and with no troublesome side
effects. But a physician's expertise extends far beyond the prescription pad.

You should be evaluated by a doctor before trying St. John's wort on
your own if you fit any of the following conditions:

- You have chronic or significant medical problems or you are under-
  going some acute illness.
- You are taking other medications.
- You have a severe depression, with suicidal tendencies, difficulty
  functioning, or deteriorating physical health as a result of depression.
- You have other psychiatric problems such as drug or alcohol problems or bipolar disorder, you have ever suffered from a schizophrenic
  or psychotic illness, or you are experiencing symptoms of dementia.
- You have had serious problems with medication in the past.
- You are uncertain about taking St. John's wort or want more information before deciding to embark on this course.

If you have any doubt that relatively mild depression is your problem,
you should seriously consider seeing a doctor before trying St. John's wort
or any other herbal remedy. Treating an illness that cannot be improved by
St. John's wort with the herb may allow your actual illness to deteriorate,

with potentially serious consequences. Also, because depression can be caused by a number of medical conditions, there is always the risk that these underlying conditions will be missed and could worsen. Possible causes could include cancer, thyroid disease, chronic pain states, anemia, chronic infectious disease, chronic obstructive pulmonary disease, and metabolic deficiencies (e.g., lack of vitamin B_{12}).

If you suspect you have more than one disorder—or you know that you do—you should also consider seeking a doctor's treatment rather than prescribing for yourself. It is quite common for depression to be associated with other psychological conditions, for example, generalized anxiety disorder (i.e., excessive worry), obsessive–compulsive disorder, and alcohol abuse. The association of more than one condition in the same person is called *comorbidity*, meaning that more than one "morbid" (i.e., abnormal) state is present at the same time. Sometimes a single treatment will be sufficient, for example, the use of an SSRI to treat depression and obsessive–compulsive disorder, since it works effectively on each of these conditions. But no studies have been done that can tell us whether this is also true for herbal remedies like St. John's wort, so you may neglect one condition while treating the other should you choose self-help over a doctor's care.

Collaborating with Your Current Doctor

Some people who are being treated for depression with a prescription medication become interested in switching to St. John's wort because they have heard so many encouraging words about its antidepressant effects. If you are among them, it may be up to you to suggest the herb to your doctor. Very few, if any, American-trained doctors learned when and how to prescribe herbal remedies such as St. John's wort during the course of their training. During the last few years, however, with the growing awareness that such treatments can help, and also in response to the public's expectations and requests, more and more doctors are becoming familiar with this treatment approach. Any medically trained doctor should quickly be able to pick up the essentials of how and when to prescribe St. John's wort. If your doctor is truly concerned about your welfare, and also recognizes the potential importance of knowledge about herbal treatments, he or she should quickly be able to find the answers to your questions.

Some doctors are still quite opposed in principle to the use of herbal treatments. However, most are open-minded, and a small but increasing number are very enthusiastic advocates. Certainly, it has been our experience from a survey that we did at Duke University that physicians are generally supportive of patients who tell them that they are taking alternative treatments. We do not know what percentage of prescribers actually recommend St. John's wort, but it is safe to say that a large number of doctors now welcome the opportunity to learn more about the place of herbal treatments, as well as to become more familiar with various brands.

If your doctor is skeptical, don't be shy about explaining any philosophical preference for herbs that you have. Practitioners of traditional medicine are now beginning to recognize the importance of respecting these leanings. In one of our panic disorder studies several years ago, we found that a normally effective drug for treating panic attacks did not work if the patient was unready to take responsibility for making the necessary changes and doing the necessary things in order to get better. In other words, for a drug to work, sometimes you are better off if you are ready to make changes and strongly want treatment. Maybe some drugs do not work as well in a reluctant patient!

If your doctor refuses to support your use of St. John's wort, be sure to ask why. If you suffer from depression-plus or your doctor feels your problem is something other than depression, St. John's wort simply may not help, or a prescription medication may have a better chance of helping you. Or your doctor simply may not be sufficiently familiar with this form of treatment. If he or she is willing to try it, then your expressing a strong personal preference for trying this treatment may make the difference. On the other hand, if your doctor is simply against using treatments of this type, it's up to you to decide whether you wish to consult another doctor.

If my doctor doesn't want to take me off my prescription, what are my options?

If you are dead set against continuing with a regular drug, make your preference crystal clear to your doctor. But also try to be open-minded so that you don't shut off other potentially effective options should your first choice of treatment fail to help you.

Your doctor and you should balance out the following considerations in choosing the best treatment for you:

- The overall evidence that a particular treatment is effective for your type of depression
- The likelihood that side effects will not be a problem
- The particular kinds of symptoms that characterize your depression

- Your philosophical preference
- Your doctor's philosophical preference
- Previous treatments you have tried
- Treatments that may have helped a close relative who with depression
- The seriousness of your depression and the urgency for responding

What this all adds up to is that in some cases an herbal treatment may be your most appropriate therapy, while in other cases an SSRI drug, perhaps a course of electroconvulsive therapy (ECT), or a course of psychotherapy may be better for you. Sometimes a combination of treatments would be the most desirable course: being on one treatment does not preclude using other types of treatment as well.

Is combining St. John's wort with another antidepressant, possibly at a lower dose than I'm currently taking, an option?

Although we have no studies to inform us about the safety and effectiveness of combining St. John's wort with other medicines, clinical practice indicates that for the most part St. John's wort can be combined safely with other drugs. The exception would be the monoamine oxidase inhibitors (MAOIs; Nardil, Parnate, Marplan, Mannerix, Aurorix), which are dangerous in combination with other drugs that have effects on serotonin, such as St. John's wort. There would be a risk of severe agitation, muscular stimulation, and increase in body temperature to a potentially lethal level.

While there is a theoretical risk that combining St. John's wort at high doses with an SSRI drug could also produce a serotonin syndrome, at regular therapeutic doses such effects are unlikely. Thus it is probably safe, under medical supervision, to take this combination. We personally have used it in our clinical practice with good effect. The most important thing is to do it in a careful and planned way. It is best to give one treatment its best shot and take a second treatment only if one drug alone has not produced an adequate response.

If you do combine these drugs, and you notice increased muscle twitching, tremor, sweating, or gastrointestinal discomfort, it is possible that the two drugs are producing increased side effects. In this case, their use should be reassessed. It is also possible that the dose of your St. John's wort does not need to be quite so high if you are already taking an SSRI drug.

If you have been taking St. John's wort and your doctor wants you to take an SSRI or another antidepressant, unless it is a MAO inhibitor, you can stop St. John's wort over a few days, and at the same time gradually begin taking the antidepressant. Similarly, if you have been on an antidepressant, and you or your doctor decides to switch you to St. John's wort, a gradual taper of the antidepressant is recommended, while a slow introduction of St. John's wort, initially perhaps 300 mg per day, with slowly increasing doses, would be reasonable.

The addition of St. John's wort to an established course of antidepressant therapy was helpful to 44-year-old Terrell, a high school football coach who had a long history of chronic worry about almost anything, as well as poor sleep, with a maximum of about four hours each night. His mood was low and his interest in everyday activities had diminished, although he did continue to be quite productive at work. There had been reduction in his sexual interest and he suffered from frequent headaches related to his depression and anxiety. A persisting and vexing symptom was recurring ideas of death and suicide, along with a general sense of blackness about the future.

Terrell had not received any medication treatment before, although he did have individual counseling following an earlier divorce. We began treating him with Serzone, but because he still had some symptoms even at the top dose of 600 mg per day, we cautiously raised the dose to 700 mg, which caused some side effects, including tingling, visual blurring, and feelings of unreality. We lowered the dose but, because he still had ongoing symptoms, added an antidepressant from a different category, Wellbutrin. This combination was of some help to Terrell, but again he complained of side effects, including stomach discomfort and some visual symptoms. Although improved, Terrell still was troubled by his persisting suicidal and fatalistic thoughts about the future. After some consideration, Terrell hesitatingly agreed to take St. John's wort as an additional medicine, with the expectation being that it might possibly provide some help without complicating the side effect picture. Despite his skepticism, after a few weeks Terrell found that the intensity of his suicidal thoughts had diminished somewhat, an effect that became more noticeable as the dose was raised from 600 mg. to 900 mg.

What Lies Ahead?

At this time we are looking forward to the results of a number of ongoing or recently completed trials of St. John's wort against placebo and/or active antidepressants, as well as studies looking at potential drug–drug interactions. Among the questions we consider important to answer are these:

- Does St. John's wort help alleviate the "blues" or "minor" depression?
- Does it have beneficial effects in anxiety or attention-deficit/hyper-activity disorder?
- Are higher doses more effective than lower doses?
- Is it effective in severe major depression?
- With which drugs does St. John's wort interact?
- Does St. John's wort prevent relapse?
- What is the utility and safety of St. John's wort in special populations, such as children, the elderly, and medically compromised individuals?
- Can St. John's wort be safely used by depressed people with other medical illnesses, and which drug and St. John's wort combinations should be avoided?

ESSENTIAL FACTS ABOUT ST. JOHN'S WORT	
Main Use	Antidepressant
Other Reported Uses	Anxiolytic (anti-anxiety), hypnotic (sleep aid), treatment for seasonal affective disorder (SAD), antibacterial, antiviral, anti-inflammatory (burn and wound healing)
When Not to Use This Herb	During pregnancy, when trying to conceive, or when breastfeeding; when taking therapeutic UV light treatments, while taking MAOI, while using cocaine, stimulants, or diet aids such as phentermine Do not self-medicate if you are taking digoxin, cyclosporine, indinavir, covmadin
Side Effects	Mild nausea, headache, sleepiness, dry mouth, constipation, itchiness, restlessness, dizziness, mania (in those at risk for bipolar disorder), sunburn (from increased sensitivity to sunlight)
When to Expect Positive Effects	After two to eight weeks of use
Common Preparation Forms	Tablets, capsules, liquid, tea, tincture, ointment (topical only), and oil (topical only, particularly aromatherapy).
Average Effective Daily Dosage	600 to 1,800 mg, standardized to 0.3 percent hypericin (1.8 to 5.4 mg hypericin), usually divided into two to three doses per day

2

Kava

Tranquility from Paradise

O, how full of briers is this working-day world!
—WILLIAM SHAKESPEARE,
As You Like It (1598–1600)

If we could rid ourselves of one modern evil, most of us would choose stress. Stress plagues up to a quarter of the U.S. workforce and possibly the same percentage of the general adult population. It wears us out, dulls our senses and our pleasures, robs us of creativity and efficiency, and literally makes us sick. It inflicts harm in many ways, both pysical and psychological.

Enter kava, a mysterious plant from the South Pacific that apparently can ease not only stress but anxiety—quickly, inexpensively, and without appreciable side effects.

If you pay attention to the news, you know that kava is currently being touted as the "great green hope" for all those who have too much work to do and too little time to do it, too many responsibilities and not enough resources, too many conflicts and too little camaraderie. What South Pacific islanders have known for 3,000 years has, in the blink of an eye, made kava one of the top-selling herbal remedies in America. Regarding kava use, Europe is way ahead of the United States—as it is with regard to herbalism in general. In Germany and other European countries kava is a government-regulated remedy that is commonly prescribed for stress, anxiety, insomnia,

> Kava is a healthy, natural way of relaxing. We don't
> need television. . . . Cares and worries disappear—
> carried away by the warm ocean wind.
> —POLYNESIAN ISLANDER
>
> There is no other plant that gives such utter
> relaxation while at the same time allowing such
> clear, penetrating mindfulness.
> —BILL BREVORT, herbalist
>
> I think kava is going to revolutionize the treatment
> of 65 million Americans who annually suffer from
> the symptoms of anxiety.
> —DR. HAROLD BLOOMFIELD,
> author of *Healing Anxiety with Herbs*

and other ills. We have been prescribing it to our own patients with great success for about three years; indeed, we have even found it personally useful as a muscle relaxant for our aching backs. Kava has been called a tranquilizer, a sedative, a narcotic, a soporific, and an analgesic. But kava has other faces as well. There is kava the ceremonial and spiritual aid, its most ancient identity. Then there is kava the social lubricant, served at "bars" throughout Polynesia and now even in some parts of the United States. Finally, there is kava the over-the-counter "dietary supplement" that a growing number of Western adults are taking to ease the stress of a demanding day, to hasten the unwinding process with a group of friends, to calm them and help them concentrate when the jitters threaten to impede success at work or at school. Observations in our research labs and clinical practice are telling us more and more about kava's powers to treat what ails us.

☙ WHAT KAVA DOES

To paint a complete picture of what this widely romanticized herb can do, we have to go back centuries to its Polynesian origins. It's difficult to say exactly where and when kava use began, though we do know the plant is native to the South Pacific and has been the stuff of legend since approximately 1000 B.C. One of the earliest kava legends conveys how the Polynesian people's belief in its potency: While staying in the Fiji Islands, a Sa-

moan girl who had married a Fijian chief observed a rat chewing on a
native plant and shortly afterward falling asleep. She then noticed that after waking up the rat moved over to chew on the root of another plant and
changed into a strong, energetic, and courageous animal. The first of these
plants was sugarcane, and the second was kava. The young girl took both
plants back to her homeland, where they grew so well that people from
other islands began to trade with the Samoans for kava.

Thanks to Polynesian seafarers, kava was carried throughout the vast
expanse of the Pacific islands, from Malaysia to Tahiti and from Hawaii to
Tonga. Some believe that kava's true native home is a few hundred miles
west of Fiji, on Vanuatu, which today remains the largest commercial pro-
ducer of the herb. Archaeological discoveries indicate that wherever it was
first used, kava became an important element in spiritual ceremonies in
many Pacific cultures over the millennia.

Today kava is probably valued most widely for its ability to produce
both relaxation and a sense of well-being. Honored as the "giver of peace-
fulness," kava purportedly calms those who take it, making them feel
friendly, outgoing, and benevolent. But unlike alcohol and other substances used to promote relaxation, kava does not reduce mental clarity or
increase aggression. Instead, it sharpens the senses and improves concentration, memory, and reaction time. One modern herbalist claims that it
not only heightens consciousness but provides greater access to the dream
state, or the subconscious.

These amazing properties made kava a mainstay of Polynesian religious ceremonies, social events, and medicine. Fiji's spiritual healers believed it connected them with a spirit force they called *Vu*, whereby they
could see into the future and feel what herbal remedies should be prescribed for their patients. Because it seems to increase amicability, kava has
also traditionally been used in conflict resolution. And today, just as centuries ago, the kava ceremony is an important part of the welcome extended
to dignitaries visiting Fiji and other Polynesian islands.

Kava remained a South Seas secret until the 1770s, when Captain
James Cook made his second voyage to the Pacific. Cook and his successors
were fascinated by kava's effects but repelled by its preparation, which
called for numerous people to chew the root and then spit the resulting liquid into a communal bowl. Perhaps stemming from the explorers' disgust
with its method of preparation, kava was not transported to Europe until
German colonists took it home with them a hundred years later.

Oddly, the herb entered the German pharmacopoeia not as a medicine for inducing relaxation and increasing mental clarity but as a treatment for gonorrhea—perhaps because sailors who suffered from gonorrhea noticed some easing of their symptoms after trying kava. However this use arose, kava remained an accepted treatment for gonorrhea in Germany until penicillin was discovered in 1928. Meanwhile, the herb was also found to be useful in treating asthma and skin disorders and as a urinary antiseptic. These uses were eventually discontinued, however, because the very high doses required caused unacceptable side effects, probably including sedation.

Early in the 20th century, German biochemical researchers, then the world leaders in this field, started to identify the active ingredients in kava. They isolated a number of chemicals, which they named *kavalactones*, that they found were responsible for the anxiety-reducing effects of kava. But it wasn't until the mid-1960s that German scientists identified the six kavalactones, out of 15, that were specifically responsible for reducing anxiety. And it took a couple more decades before a full double-blind placebo-controlled study produced reliable data on kava's effects.

For us, kava was an unknown quantity until a doctor friend in Germany mentioned that it was a hot-selling item manufactured by a major pharmaceutical firm and one of the most popular treatments for anxiety and stress in her country. Our curiosity was piqued and we began to investigate further. What was it? Where could it be found in the United States? How could it be used? Would it work as well as regular treatments for anxiety? Would it be a credible replacement for commonly prescribed drugs?

A growing body of research indicates that kava can indeed be a valuable alternative to prescription drugs for those who suffer from mild to moderate anxiety. This claim is supported by our own clinical practice. We have seen kava induce a pleasant state of calm, contentment, and unconcern about worries, just as the Polynesians have always described. A few of our patients have reported that kava makes them feel more sociable and promotes conversation. We have also noticed that kava seems to increase people's sensitivity to sound and light and to magnify their powers of attention and concentration. Kava has reduced pain and increased muscle relaxation in the back and joints, and it has also induced sleep. Some of our patients like kava for its lack of side effects, others for how quickly it has helped them.

Ken, a 68-year-old retired air traffic controller, had experienced lifelong tension, worry, and distressing stomach symptoms whenever he felt under pressure. He often found himself distractible and unable to concentrate, for example, when reading or playing cards. He had never been treated for anxiety before, but on 210 mg of kavalactones per day, he found that for the first time in his life he was able to relax and enjoy his card games with full concentration. "Now I know what it is like for other, 'normal' people. I could never understand how my wife was able to sit down and relax. Now I can do it," he reported.

Tamika, a 32-year-old administrator, reported that kava helped her deal with many stresses at work and in her personal life as she went through a divorce by helping her "focus on the task and not on my distress."

Luther, a 59-year-old truck driver, found kava so effective in relieving stress that he recommended it to his wife. "She is much less tense now," he says. "She doesn't chew my head off from the irritability and snappiness she used to have."

Natasha, a 35-year-old-nurse who had always been prone to excessive worry, started taking kava when she felt overwhelmed by anxiety over the upcoming closing on her new home. As the closing drew near, she told us, "I don't know what there was to worry about so much. Now I'm looking forward to it!"

Obviously kava has come a long way from its ancient use as a mood-altering and mind-expanding ritual drug. But the herb's metamorphosis into an herbal remedy for stress and anxiety is not as great a leap as it may at first look. Consider the known benefits of kava against the common symptoms of anxiety: tranquility and relaxation instead of excessive worry, amiability and gregariousness in place of grouchiness and tension, alertness and sharp attention instead of the dulled decision making and poor concentration that results from nervousness. This description is an oversimplified sketch, but it illustrates why researchers in this century started looking at kava's potential to treat anxiety.

How did we go from treating anxiety with kava to treating stress with the herb? Anxiety generally causes us either to avoid situations that we read as stressful or to fret and worry constantly. When a remedy like kava relaxes us, those anxiety-producing situations might seem less stressful, heading off some of the worry, fear, and avoidance they usually stimulate. In other words, kava may make us feel less anxious and less stressed out in one fell swoop. But those who first tried using kava to ease stress were probably moved mainly by the similarity between symptoms of stress and the symptoms of anxiety (see Table 6).

The main differences between anxiety and stress lie in the areas of du-

Table 6. Anxiety versus Stress: Similarity of Symptoms

	Anxiety disorder	Stress
Physical symptoms		
Headaches	Yes	Yes
Back pain	Yes	Yes
Fatigue	Yes	Yes
Poor sexual functioning	Yes	Yes
Poor sleep	Yes	Yes
Stomach problems	Yes	Yes
Mood/mental symptoms		
Anxious	Yes	Yes
Irritable	Yes	Yes
Worried	Yes	Yes
Distractible	Yes	Yes
Behaviors		
Declining work productivity	Yes	Yes
Strained relationships	Yes	Yes
Increased eating, or use of alcohol	Yes	Yes

ration and number of symptoms, potential impairment level, extent of distress, and coherence of symptoms. In other words, stress and anxiety overlap a great deal, but anxiety is more readily recognizable as a cluster of co-occuring symptoms that make it more difficult for an individual to function normally.

These distinctions may be more meaningful to doctors than to their patients, however. When you're the one who's suffering the symptoms, it can be very easy to confuse the two conditions. Emilio, a native of South America and the son of a lawyer, came to the United States with his wife and three children to complete his doctoral studies. At first he did very well at his job as a statistical analyst for a software company. Before long, however, his moodiness, tardiness, and isolation led to several confrontations with his supervisor, who grew increasingly unhappy with Emilio's work.

Emilio believed all of his problems, including regular headaches, stemmed from stress, but on his wife's insistence he came to see us. After giving him a detailed evaluation, we told Emilio that we thought his real problem was a form of anxiety called *social phobia*. We explained that his isolation and moodiness were rooted in his extreme fear of suffering embarrassment and humiliation. We started Emilio on Zoloft (sertraline), one of the newer generation antidepressants, which produce few side effects and are often effective for anxiety as well as depression. Emilio did not like the increased appetite and accompanying weight gain that came were the side effects of this drug's lessening of his anxiety. Emilio opted next for a nonmedication approach and began cognitive therapy and biofeedback. These treatments helped him somewhat, but Emilio was still quite tense in both social and work situations. Finally we suggested that kava might be helpful for him. After starting a regular dose of three 210-mg capsules per day, Emilio reported feeling much more relaxed and less self-conscious. He began to get along better with his coworkers, stopped arriving late for work, and no longer lost himself in worry about losing his job.

Emilio's case had a happy ending, but it raises some interesting issues that have accompanied the rise in popularity of herbal remedies. On the one hand, the ready availability and perceived harmlessness of herbs have led many people to self-treat mild disorders that would have gone untreated in the past. That's a good thing. On the other hand, easy access to herbal remedies may divert some people to self-treatment when a doctor's care would serve them better. Disinclined toward seeking help as he was, if Emilio had simply bought some kava after his wife had read about it, tried the dose recommended on the label, and found it to be of little help, he may have given up, unaware that he was taking far too little to help him.

On the other side of the coin are people whose experience has made them such highly satisfied customers of kava that they will believe any claim made for it. Despite the fact that there is virtually no scientific evidence to support these claims, various sources have advocated kava for treating everything from fungal infections to high blood pressure, from migraine headaches to gout to whooping cough. It's been called a diuretic, an anti-inflammatory, a bronchial agent, and even an aphrodisiac.

In truth, there is still an awful lot that we don't know about what kava does. Kava has not yet been studied as systematically as St. John's wort and ginkgo, which means we need a lot more hard science to confirm or refute what legend and anecdote have told us about kava's healing powers. We also don't know everything we need to know about its other powers. As history has shown, many "feel good" substances eventually reveal a darker side. Until scientists systematically accumulate much more data on the herb, we can't be sure that kava doesn't have a "down side" of its own, like those revealed for alcohol, tobacco, and other widely used substances. For now we're operating with voids in our knowledge in many areas, including these important questions regarding what kava does:

- How can we tell whether kava is likely to help any individual person?
- What symptoms are appropriately treated by kava?
- Does kava have the same effects when taken over the long term as it does when taken over the short term?
- What is the risk of abuse or dependence?
- Do kava's effects change when it is combined with other medicines?
- Does it work the same way for occasional stress relief as it does in treating diagnosable anxiety?

How quickly we gain answers to these questions depends on how rapidly case histories are accumulated and reported by clinicians and how much additional research is undertaken. Check the Resources section at the back of this book for ways to keep up with information from new studies, which generally are not publicized until researchers present their findings at meetings or publish them in journals. Throughout the rest of this chapter we will share the findings of scientific studies done to date.

From everything I've read, kava sounds like the latest legal recreational drug. Which is it, a legitimate herbal remedy or just another alternative to liquor?

Your confusion is understandable. Serious herbalists have been touting kava as a panacea for the symptoms of stress, but lots of kava enthusiasts have spread the word on TV and the Internet, in magazines and newsletters, that kava is the "feel good" party refreshment for the new millennium. But while kava and alcohol share similar social uses, *it would be a serious mistake to think of kava as just another alcohol substitute.* Not only does kava differ from alcohol in many important ways, but we just don't know enough about it yet to understand all of the potential dangers associated with its recreational use. So, as kava bars begin to spread eastward from the West Coast—rather like latter-day Starbucks coffee franchises—we advise you to treat kava cautiously and responsibly, as you would alcohol.

Remember, above all, that kava is a pharmacologically active drug, which means its use is not without risk. Kava can be sedating; as the dose increases, it can slow your reaction time and leave you feeling unsteady, clumsy, and "washed out." Your driving ability can be impaired. So far the research shows that the danger may be minimal unless substantial doses are ingested, but we don't know enough yet about how kava's effects vary from individual to individual to be sure that anyone imbibing kava at a "bar" will not end up impaired and a danger to himself and others. While it doesn't seem to do so in moderate therapeutic quantities, kava *may* increase the effects of other drugs and of alcohol. The reverse is also true: other drugs can increase the effects of kava. At very high doses, and with long-term use, kava can impair physical health.

Even if you believe you are being careful regarding how much kava you take for recreational purposes, you can't be sure about the potency of the kava preparations served at bars or parties. In other words, you may decide to have "just one," but that "one" may not be the equivalent of the light beer that you expected but instead pack the punch of a triple martini!

For all of these reasons, we do not endorse the recreational use of kava. We realize, however, that this is a choice that each person is free to make. As with many medicines, kava can affect different individuals in different ways, and not everyone will like the feeling they get from it. Rafael, a 36-year-old auto mechanic from Mexico, had taken kava for nervous tension but stopped it after a few days because it made him feel sluggish, depressed, and "washed out." He also didn't like the "spaced-out" feeling he experienced.

During a really tough period last year I tried a tablet that was a combination of kava and St. John's wort, hoping that it might help me shake off the blues, the sleeplessness, the irritability, and the general uneasiness I was feeling. It ended up making me feel really weird, sort of spacy and high in a dizzy way, so I didn't try it again. Does this mean that what I was feeling wasn't stress after all?

That's extremely difficult to tell without a lot more information. First of all, the reaction you had may have been a product of how much active ingredient of each herb was in the pill you took, the proportion of kava to St. John's wort, or a number of other factors. It's also possible that you are one of the people who doesn't like the feeling that kava imparts. Either way, the side effects of this preparation obviously outweighed any benefits. Since you didn't like how you felt after taking one pill, it's hard to say whether you actually received any stress-reducing benefits. Since you don't report feeling less stress, we assume you did not respond to the remedy, and that's a different issue from experiencing side effects. Nonresponse does not necessarily mean you're not suffering from stress. Maybe kava just isn't the right remedy for your stress symptoms. But the possibility that stress isn't really what's bothering you is why it can be so important to understand what's wrong before trying various solutions. Let's look at what we know about stress compared to what we know about anxiety and see how kava fits in with treatment of each.

Kava for Stress: A Welcome Relief

You probably believe you know exactly what stress feels like. Few of us today have managed to escape the burned-out, wrung-out, tense, on-the-edge feelings that stress imposes. But stress is a complicated state, with a wide variety of symptoms. You may not recognize some symptoms you're suffering as signs of stress, or you may, as Emilio did, attribute certain symptoms to stress when something else is at work. Either error can make it hard for you to manage your own care. To get an idea of whether you are suffering from stress, review the following list. But remember that these symptoms and behaviors can be caused by a number of other problems, including anxiety and the medical conditions listed on page 114.

Physically, people under stress may experience headaches, neck stiffness, upper or lower back pain, general muscle fatigue, unsatisfactory sexual functioning, broken sleep, excessive sleep, and/or stomach problems. Moreover, medical disorders such as asthma, migraine, irritable bowel syndrome, peptic ulcer, and high blood pressure can be initiated or made worse by stress.

- Stress changes the way you feel and can make you anxious, irritable, moody, worried, and distractible. It saps energy and motivation and can leave you with less than normal initiative.
- If you're under stress, you may alter your behavior patterns, for example, by using recreational drugs, alcohol, or cigarettes excessively, or by changing your eating habits. Your work performance may also suffer; it is not unusual for a person under great stress to miss time from work.
- High stress often leads to strained relationships. You may have frequent arguments with others, withdraw or isolate yourself, begin an extramarital affair, or avoid your usual social or community activities.

Essentially, stress is the result of not having adjusted satisfactorily to an emotional or physical event. Typical stressful events include increased job pressure, serious illness, divorce, a death in the family, financial problems, responsibility for aging parents, raising a family single-handedly, working more than one job to make ends meet, or—as is so common today—a combination of several of these. Events that are stressful tend to be unpredictable and uncontrollable, leaving us feeling powerless and unprepared and powerless. When many elements in our lives seem to fit this description, we end up feeling as if we're in a constant state of alert. As a result of this heightened state, our body suffers physical symptoms and emotional change, accompanied by alterations in behavior and/or relationships. When these stressful events persist, and we fail to adapt to them, the effects of stress take a greater and greater toll. That's why it's so important to know what you are dealing with and to take steps now to reduce stress.

Measuring Your Stress

How do you know when it's time to do something about stress rather than accept it as an inevitable fact of modern life? Is it possible to be suffering damage from stress without being aware of it? Because what is stressful for one person may not be stressful for another, the best way to measure stress is to determine how severely it is impairing your daily activity and your overall sense of well-being. Fill in the following chart to help gauge your current stress level.

If your total score indicates moderate or severe stress, you should consider treatment. Use this chart to target key symptoms now and then fill it in again several times during treatment to monitor your progress. If your scores remain the same, shifting to another treatment option would be wise.

Sometimes stress is sneaky. You may not feel all that bad, or the effects of the stress *can* build so gradually that you aren't really aware that you're suffering a great deal of stress. If your score on the stress chart surprises you, you may be suffering the hidden effects of stress.

You may also be suffering the natural effects of a stressful event. In 1967 Drs. Thomas Holmes and Richard Rahe at the University of Washington in Seattle published a scale in which they rated the degree to which particular events were stressful or, more precisely, the degree to which the burden of readjustment was heaviest. Their scale consisted of 43 events, headed by death of a spouse (rated as 100). In second, third, fourth, and

Stress Self-Assessment

Stresses in my life are affecting me in the following ways:

	Not at all 0	A little 1	Quite a bit 2	Very much 3
I am impatient	☐	☐	☐	☐
I have headaches	☐	☐	☐	☐
My sleep is poor	☐	☐	☐	☐
I get irritable at others	☐	☐	☐	☐
I feel overwhelmed	☐	☐	☐	☐
It feels like I have no control over things	☐	☐	☐	☐
It is hard to relax	☐	☐	☐	☐
My muscles feel tight	☐	☐	☐	☐

Scores of	0–8	=	None to mild symptoms
	9–16	=	Moderate symptoms
	17–24	=	Severe symptoms

fifth places were divorce (73), marital separation (65), jail term (63), and death of a close family member (63). At the bottom of the scale were events like vacation (13), Christmas holidays (12), and minor violations of the law (11). This scale has been widely used and can be found in the *Journal of Psychosomatic Research*. If you can link your stress to a recent event, your stress may fade on its own as the event recedes into the past.

What to Do When Stress Is a Problem

Now that you know whether stress is hurting you, what can you do about it?

Hundreds of books and articles have been written about how to beat stress. Workshops and seminars that train people in managing—if not conquering—stress are offered by organizations ranging from corporations to religious institutions to health care facilities to community centers. The advice they offer boils down to two basic rules (1) reduce the number of stressful elements in your life and (2) reduce the impact of stressful events on you. If you can't follow rule 1—by changing jobs, getting help with a sick family member, and so on—you can follow rule 2 by trying one of the stress-reducing methods that have proved effective for many people.

Deep breathing, muscle relaxation, and meditation are all good ways to bring tranquility to your life. Numerous books on these techniques can be found at your local library. You can use all three of these simple techniques at any time to counteract anxiety or stress that strikes suddenly and also on a regular basis to prevent a buildup of tension and worry. Adding regular exercise to your daily routine has a similar effect.

Laughter is a well-known antidote for distress, as is communing with nature. As oversimplified as it may sound, reaching out to others cuts stress and tension for many people. Try sharing your cares with a friend rather than brooding over them and look for community, church, and volunteer activities to get involved in. Find a hobby you enjoy to distract you from the day's worries and avoid relying on alcohol, caffeine, or tobacco to deal with your stress.

Kava: One Answer to Stress

As of this writing, the best evidence we have that kava can be an answer to everyday stress comes from a study conducted by Nirbhay Singh and his colleagues (1998) in Richmond, Virginia, that has been presented at a scientific meeting but not yet published. Comparatively healthy individuals who were dealing with daily stress were given either 240 mg of kavalactones or placebo for four weeks. The results showed quite clearly that daily stress due to interpersonal problems, personal competency, everyday hassles, and other stressors was significantly reduced in those who took the active treatment (kava). In addition, general levels of high anxiety were significantly reduced in those taking kava. Singh et al. reported that kava did not help *trait anxiety*, the enduring tendency of a person to easily get anxious. Of course, it is possible that a longer course of treatment might have been helpful even in this regard.

Besides this study, we have anecdotal reports from South Pacific islanders over many centuries, recent clinical observations in Germany, and our own clinical practice to attest to the fact that kava can certainly help to reduce the intensity of stress symptoms and promote a more focused ability to cope with daily problems. We can also extrapolate from several controlled studies that have shown kava to be effective in controlling anxiety.

Clinicians both in Europe and in the United States are prescribing kava for stress in the hope that the herb will ease the symptoms that stress shares with anxiety. What remains to be determined, scientifically and clinically, is exactly when, how, and to what extent kava helps relieve stress.

Is kava best for mild or for severe stress?

Kava can help *all* levels of stress and anxiety. The subjects in the Singh et al. study were in the top 33 percent of the population for severity of daily stress symptoms, and kava proved useful to them. But, as with any treatment, kava's effectiveness is least certain in the most severe cases. The more distress and discomfort stress causes you, and the more your life is impaired—at work, in your personal relationships, and so on—the more likely it is that you will need more than over-the-counter kava to return you to normal functioning and contentment. But kava certainly may still play a role in a treatment plan that incorporates psychotherapy and other options.

Should I take kava just when I feel like I'm really stressed out or all the time, as a preventive measure?

A lot depends on your circumstances. Many people take kava at the end of a particularly stressful day, when they find it hard to relax. But on run-of-the mill days, these same people find that a workout at the gym, a movie with a friend, or a walk in the woods may be all they need to unwind. For occasional periods of high tension, stress, or worry, you too might take kava as needed and stop taking it once the symptoms of stress have gone away.

If your stresses are continuous, you might want to take kava every day to avoid the ups and downs of periodic use. There is no point in waiting for the symptoms to reappear before taking kava if you are quite certain that they will in fact reappear as long as the stressor exists.

Do I have to think far ahead? What if I suddenly feel stressed out right before I have to make an important presentation? Will kava work right away?

Kava can work quickly, even within a few hours. So, if you have a big presentation to give, or an important interview, for example, taking one or two kava capsules a few hours beforehand might work to reduce your stress. Alternatively, you could take it when you go to bed the night before your presentation, enjoy a refreshing night's sleep, and wake in a good frame of mind for your presentation.

If I start taking kava at the first sign of stress, won't I lose my "edge"?

One of the first people to study the stress response, Dr. Hans Selye, referred to it as "the rate of wear and tear in the body." Wear and tear doesn't sound particularly beneficial, but some stress can be good for us. Muscles that are never stressed atrophy and weaken, whereas those that are "stressed" become strong. Sometimes, stressful experiences can strengthen us and offer important possibilities of growth. We often hear about tales of bravery and comradeship under the extreme stress of war. Perhaps those are a product of the state of alertness that accompanies stress. So we suppose if you never experience stress and are never on alert, you might not have that "edge." The key, in our opinion, is to take kava only for relief of distressing or interfering symptoms of stress. Kava can be taken for mild or moderate stress if you find it beneficial, but if you have no symptoms of stress, just don't take it. Obviously, then, we don't endorse any "recreational use"; we recommend kava only for legitimate symptoms.

My therapist says I'm still suffering from the stress of a terrible car accident I was in several years ago. Can kava help me get over this?

One special kind of stress that needs to be understood separately is *traumatic stress*. Traumatic stress is a particular kind of reaction to loss of life, serious physical injury, or serious threats to one's physical safety or integrity. Events of this type include sexual assault, violent criminal assault, military combat, serious accident or other injury, natural disaster like a flood or hurricane, and other events such as fire, near drowning, and so forth. Just as with any stress, traumatic stress produces an emotional response in its victims. In this case, however, the response is much more intense and very negative, being characterized by fear, horror, or helplessness.

Following traumatic stress, about one in five women or one in 10 men will develop a condition called *posttraumatic stress disorder* (PTSD), which consists of well-recognized symptoms and can last for many years. The symptoms are grouped into intrusive experiences (e.g., memories, flashbacks, nightmares of the event), avoidance of anything that reminds the individual of the trauma, numbing of emotion, and increased arousal (e.g., poor concentration, poor sleep, increased irritability, greater degree of star- tle to unexpected sounds, and a general watchfulness). As you'll see on page 115, PTSD is actually considered an anxiety disorder.

While we know that kava can be helpful for everyday stress, we have no information at all about whether it is useful in treating PTSD.

How do I know whether it would be better for me to take kava or to use one of the nonmedicinal stress-relieving methods, like yoga or hiking?

The most successful forms of stress relief vary from one person to another. In some cases, an integrated approach is best. Thus kava may well be an im- portant component of a treatment plan that also includes, for example, meditation and regular exercise. Others may find that regular use of yoga is sufficient, and still others will benefit sufficiently from simply taking kava from time to time. Trial and error is really the only way to find out what is best for you. We suggest that you start out with the treatment that seems most comfortable for you and then progress to the others if your first trials are not satisfactory.

Other herbal remedies are said to relieve stress too. How do I know kava is the best one for me?

Several herbal remedies have been used to relieve symptoms of stress and anxiety. Unfortunately, there is precious little useful scientific data attest- ing to these effects.

Valerian, the subject of Chapter 4, was used to treat so many people who had suffered shell shock (or PTSD) during World War I that supplies of high-grade material were exhausted. However, we have not been able to locate references that describe its effects and/or whether it really did help. A recent study by Dressing et al. (1996) of 48 patients with insomnia found that valerian reduced symptoms of anxiety. This could be related to the ability of valerian to act via a chemical compound called *gamma amino- butyric acid* (GABA), a major inhibitory ("calming") neurochemical in the brain.

St. John's wort, which affects both serotonin and GABA, also has anxiolytic (anxiety-reducing) effects. Although we lack controlled studies, and thus scientific proof, we have been struck by the ability of this remedy to reduce phobic fears such as fear of flying and fear of water. It also helps to remove or lessen the amount of general worry in people's lives.

Although passionflower (*Passiflora incarnata*) and hops (*Humulus lupus*) have been used in the past for stress, "nerves," and anxiety, we have no direct experience with their use. They are, however, indicated in Germany for the treatment of these disorders. Hops, for example, are indicated for restlessness, anxiety, and sleep disturbance at a single dose of 0.5 grams. There are no known contraindications or side effects. (The word *hops* calls to mind the production of beer. However, hops as an herbal remedy does not contain alcohol, as they are not fermented. We suspect that, to the extent that beer may be calming, it is the result of its alcohol content and not its hops flavoring.) Passionflower, at a daily dose of 4 to 8 grams, is indicated for nervous restlessness. No contraindications or side effects are listed. Passionflower was listed in the U.S. National Formulary before being dropped in 1936. The FDA continued to recognize it as an over-the-counter sedative and sleep aid before withdrawing its approval in 1978, due to lack of evidence for efficacy.

At the present time, based on available evidence, we consider kava the herb that is best established and the likely first choice in the herbal treatment of stress or anxiety.

For more severe states of anxiety (PTSD, severe generalized anxiety disorder, obsessive–compulsive disorder, and severe social phobia) we do not regard kava as a first-choice treatment, however, nor do we know yet whether it is effective.

What about multiherb preparations including kava?

No such combinations are mentioned in the German Commission E monograph, and we have no reason to believe such products are more effective or any safer. It's always harder to discern the effectiveness of any component in a multiherb preparation. We recommend sticking to plain kava, which is the only product for which we have any reliable data.

Kava reduced my stress only a little bit. What should I do?

You have several options:

- Try adding one of the other stress relief methods along with kava (see pages 103 and 107). An integrated approach works best for many people.

- Try increasing the dose of kava (see pages 135 and 136). You may not be taking enough.
- See a doctor. Your symptoms may be too severe for kava alone, or something other than stress and anxiety may be causing them.

Kava as a Remedy for Anxiety

We've all felt anxiety at some time or another, whether prompted by fear of failure in the middle of the bar exam, worry about the safety of a young child on her first trip away from home, or overwhelming stage fright before a speech. Thankfully, these states usually pass. But sometimes they never quite leave us. We're always on alert, ready for the worst to happen, unwilling and perhaps eventually even unable to put ourselves in the situations that make our heart beat faster, our breath come quicker, and our skin heat up or chill down without regard to the ambient temperature. Anxiety takes many forms, but in general it makes us avoid the circumstances that cause us fear and discomfort. We might put off dental visits, resign ourselves to low-level jobs because they don't require presentations in front of groups, spend excessive time and money running to the doctor, or lead lives of solitude to escape potential social embarrassment. We may talk ourselves out of all kinds of opportunities for fulfillment and happiness by paralyzing ourselves with "what-ifs."

Anxiety disorders as defined by psychiatrists are well-recognized groupings of symptoms centering on excessive worry, fear, panic, avoidance, or obsessions and compulsions. To be diagnosed with an anxiety disorder your everyday functioning would have to be impaired or your anxiety would have to cause you excessive levels of distress. But there are lesser degrees of anxiety—known as subclinical anxiety—that would not meet the criteria for a diagnosis of an anxiety disorder yet still cause much damage to people's lives. Perhaps you have an extremely shy friend who would spend every weekend at home in front of the TV if you didn't coax her out of the house now and then. Or you have a relative whose worries about minutiae put a damper on every family gathering. Or you know a neighbor whose exaggerated fears about germs keep her child from attending birthday parties, field trips, and day camps. And almost all of us know someone who has become "obsessed" with worry or immersed in angst over some aspect of life: the smart young corporate manager who can't stop talking about work, the middle-aged employee who is terrified of ending up destitute in his old age, the complainer who thinks she never gets her fair share, or the hyper-senstive person who has to rehash every conversation in his mind, search-ing for nuances of insult. Mild anxiety could be at the root of all such behavior. Though relatively gentle remedies like kava could possibly make a world of difference for such anxiety sufferers, most people never seek help.

Burt is typical of the many people in the world who suffer from worry that would probably be considered subclinical anxiety or a severe "stress re-action." A 34-year-old restaurant manager, Burt could hardly bear up to the pressures he faced at work every day. From the waiter who never showed up on time to the constant complaints of customers, Burt felt overwhelmed by problems that he seemed unable to solve. He began to lose himself in worry about being fired and spent perhaps as much as 30 percent of his time wor-rying and berating himself for being a failure.

Burt managed to get through his workday, but he practically crawled home at closing time, usually with a pounding headache. He often poured himself a couple of stiff drinks and fell into bed without eating, only to find himself staring at the ceiling, lost in ruminations over how he would ever get another job if he lost this one.

One night, desperate to distract himself long enough to get sleepy, Burt pored through the daily paper and discovered an article about kava. He bought a bottle of capsules the next day. After two weeks on four cap-sules a day he felt much better. He was starting to sleep a full seven hours daily, and his workday was less and less likely to be interrupted by attacks of anxiety whenever a little problem arose at the restaurant.

Ultimately Burt fired his constantly tardy waiter and realized that the number and degree of his customers' complaints was no greater than it had ever been. What had been driving him crazy with worry was just a normal part of business.

Kava did not "cure" Burt. If he had seen a psychologist or a psychia-trist, he would undoubtedly have learned through an evaluation that he had always tended toward excessive worry. Kava relaxed him and cleared his mind just enough to help him realize that most of his discomfort lay in the way he was interpreting events. On the advice of a friend, he began to take books out of the library on perceptions and beliefs, beginning his own self-help cognitive-behavorial therapy. Understanding that his perception of events could be controlled rather than allowed to control him was Burt's long-term savior, but without kava he might never have taken the neces-sary steps toward ending a life of worry.

Joanna's anxiety was more specific. A 20-year-old college sophomore, she was living the life of a bright, successful student and athlete with plenty of friends, except for one cloud on her horizon: whenever she had to give a class presentation, she would freeze up, blush, get trembly, and experience terrible palpitations of her heart, which beat so hard she felt as though it would burst out of her chest. For the two days before any such presentation she would be unable to sleep, which certainly didn't add to her performance. Encouraged by a roommate, Joanna decided to take kava, three capsules a day, for two or three days before her next presentation. Kava appeared to help her sleep well and, on the day of the event, enabled her to give her speech without any more fear and discomfort than most people would feel. With other relaxation techniques and/or cognitive-behavioral therapy, Joanna could probably learn to adjust her beliefs and therefore her fears about public speaking. But these methods take time, and while she's working with them she can prevent her stage fright from ruining her life by using kava to help her relax.

Anxiety is not all bad, any more than stress is all bad. In the early part of the 20th century, two psychologists, Drs. Yerkes and Dodson, came up with what is now called the *Yerkes–Dodson law*, which relates the amount of anxiety to a person's performance. Without any question, having a limited degree of anxiety helps prepare us for situations that call for peak performance or best response. If you are walking across the road and a car comes toward you without showing any signs of stopping, you are likely to quickly take appropriate action, for example, by running out of the way immediately. This kind of "fight-or-flight" response requires an increased level of alertness, without which you would put yourself in danger. Likewise, if you have to give a speech or a presentation, you will almost certainly have some anxiety ahead of time, which may motivate you to get well prepared. On the other hand, if you have excessive levels of anxiety, your mind will be distracted, your body will be up in arms, and you will have a variety of troublesome symptoms like heart palpitations, sweating, inattentiveness, and shaking.

The Yerkes–Dodson law as depicted in Figure 1, shows this relationship. Some anxiety is appropriate and adaptive, but too much anxiety is inappropriate, distressing, and maladaptive. If your anxiety level falls on the right side of the curve, you need to figure out ways to bring yourself back to the left side—that is, to reduce your level of anxiety—to maximize your performance in all that you do.

Finding the "right" level of stress or anxiety is no mean feat. What

Performance

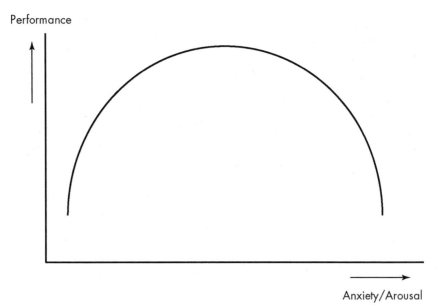

Anxiety/Arousal

Figure 1. Relationship between levels of anxiety and performance (Yerkes–Dodson law).

may at first feel energizing and invigorating may over time sap your strength and exhaust your creativity, and you may not notice the shift right away. You may want to step back and ask yourself the following questions to determine whether anxiety is beginning to harm your life:

- Do I feel distressed by my anxiety level or the duration of my heightened alertness?
- Am I avoiding situations that cause me anxiety?
- Does my life or any area of it seem diminished or less than I'd like it to be because of stress anxiety?

If you can answer Yes to any of these questions, you might consider self-treating your anxiety, perhaps with kava. If you were to seek a professional evaluation, the professional you consult might well rate your anxiety using the Hamilton Anxiety Scale (Hamilton, 1959), reproduced below. Although the Hamilton scale is designed to be used by an interviewer, you could rate yourself on this scale as a rough guide to how debilitating your anxiety may be.

Hamilton Anxiety Scale (Hamilton, 1959)

Each item is rated from 0 to 4.

0	1	2	3	4
Absent	Mild	Moderate	Severe	Extremely severe
	(less than 50% of the time or cause little interference)	(more than 50% of the time or cause moderate interference)	(substantial or marked interference more than 50% of the time)	(as bad as could be, very disabling)

☐ Anxious mood (worry, irritability, apprehensiveness)

☐ Tension (startle, crying, fatigue, trembling, unable to relax, restlessness)

☐ Phobic fear (such as of strangers, being alone, animals, traffic, crowds, other situations)

☐ Insomnia (difficulty falling or staying asleep, disturbing dreams, tired on waking)

☐ Poor concentration or memory

☐ Depression (low mood, low interest, less pleasure, waking early)

☐ Muscle symptoms (aches, stiffness, pain, jerks, grinding teeth, unsteady voice)

☐ Sensory symptoms (ringing in ears, blurred vision, hot or cold flashes, weakness, tingling)

☐ Heart symptoms (racing, skipping, pounding, chest pain, fainting feelings)

☐ Respiratory symptoms (trouble breathing, chest pressure, choking, sighing, can't catch breath)

☐ Abdominal symptoms (stomach pain, nausea, rumbling, heartburn, loose bowels, constipation, sinking feeling)

☐ Urinary and sexual symptoms (frequent or urgent urination, lower sexual desire, orgasm problems, erectile problems, premature ejaculation)

☐ Autonomic symptoms (flushing, paleness, lightheadedness, headaches, goose bumps, sweating)

☐ Restlessness

From Hamilton, M. (1959). The assessment of anxiety states by rating. *The British Journal of Medical Psychology, 32* 50–55. © The British Psychological Society.

A score of 0 to 10 reflects minimal to mild anxiety, for which self-treatment would be appropriate. A score in the range of 11 to 20 would reflect mild to moderate anxiety. Self-treatment may work in this range, but professional help may be needed, especially if a course of self-help has failed or if symptoms are interfering with your life. Scores above 20 reflect moderate to severe anxiety and would indicate that a professional opinion is advisable.

When Something Else Might Be Causing Your Anxiety

Before considering self-treatment, be aware that other problems could be causing your anxiety. Your symptoms could be caused by depression, drug withdrawal, or a medical condition. If you have already been diagnosed with one of the following conditions, it could be causing anxiety along with other symptoms:

Chronic obstructive pulmonary disease (emphysema)
Coronary artery disease (heart disease)
Hyperthyroidism (or other active thyroid condition)
Pheochromocytoma (an adrenal gland tumor)
Hypoglycemia (low blood sugar)
Vertigo
Menopause
Epilepsy (seizure disorder)

Also, a number of different drugs can give rise to symptoms of anxiety, including alcohol, stimulants (e.g., cocaine), speed, yohimbine (an aphrodisiac), caffeine, antihistamines, and steroids.

Do You Have an Anxiety Disorder?

More severe anxiety is divided into a number of disorders. A fair amount is known about each of the different anxiety disorders, what causes them, what their course is likely to be over time, what complications can develop, and what treatments work. How can you determine whether you're suffering from an anxiety disorder? Start with the checklist on page 115.

If you experience the following symptoms persistently (e.g., for several months and most of the time) and they cause you distress or limit your ability to function, you may have a clinical anxiety disorder.

If you answered Yes to any of these, you may have an anxiety disorder, and we recommend that you consider having a professional evaluation. Less than 30 percent of the people whose symptoms would qualify them for a diagnosis of one of the anxiety disorders according to an accepted convention such as the *Diagnostic and Statistical Manual of Mental Disorders*, fourth edition (DSM-IV), ever receive the treatment they need. Our checklist is, of course, oversimplified. It is not intended to be used for self-diagnosis but to

	No	Yes

Generalized anxiety disorder (GAD)

Worry, which is hard to control, more days than not for at least six months. ☐ ☐

Posttraumatic stress disorder (PTSD)

Persistent reexperiencing in memory or dreams of a terrifying experience which resulted in actual or threatened death or injury. ☐ ☐

Obsessive–compulsive disorder (OCD)

Recurring and often senseless thoughts or impulses that you cannot get out of your mind, or repetitive behaviors (like cleaning or checking) that you feel driven to perform. ☐ ☐

Social phobia

Marked and persistent fear of embarrassment or scrutiny in performance situations, or when meeting strangers or authority figures. ☐ ☐

Panic disorder

Episodes of intense fear or discomfort (panic), starting abruptly and reaching a peak within 10 minutes, accompanied by distressing physical symptoms (e.g., palpitations, dizziness, faintness). Fearful avoidance of situations may develop (agoraphobia). ☐ ☐

give you an initial idea of whether you might have an anxiety disorder. If you think you do, only a professional will be able to help you figure out which type of anxiety disorder you may have and what to do about it.

Ruth is a 57-year-old homemaker who once had a part-time job as an office assistant/receptionist in a dental practice but had to quit after a few months because of her nervousness. She couldn't shake fearful thoughts that she would make a serious mistake and fail at her job. When she wasn't consumed by fear over her occupational shortcomings, Ruth was practically drowning in anxiety over her health. Every headache heralded a possible brain tumor, every pimple a skin cancer. Ruth couldn't sleep. In fact, she no longer even tried to go to sleep. She just roamed around her house, wringing her hands, or flipped from channel to channel on late-night TV. Naturally she was exhausted, unable to complete the simplest of tasks during the day, and prone to bursting into tears at the slightest frustration.

Ruth's family doctor diagnosed her with generalized anxiety disorder and prescribed first Buspar (buspirone), then Xanax (alprazolam), and finally Prozac. Each drug helped her to some degree, but side effects always caused new problems. At the prompting of her daughter, Ruth asked her doctor about kava. He was supportive and suggested a dose of 210 mg of kavalactones per day. After three weeks, Ruth felt much more relaxed, more able to concentrate ("I balanced the checkbook in one sitting!" she exclaimed), and was sleeping better. Moreover, she reported no side effects.

Ruth still did not feel confident enough to return to work, but she did begin to volunteer at the local hospital. Her volunteer work provided her with some welcome social outlets and gave her a sense of contributing to the welfare of others in need.

Trisha was unspeakably shy. A 32-year-old computer programmer, she performed brilliantly at a job that required very little human contact, but outside of work she was extremely isolated. She shunned social events, avoided shopping, and wouldn't go to church for fear people would see her and she would blush. She found it impossible to eat in public lest she spill her food in front of others. Shy since childhood, Trisha could count on one hand the number of dates she had had. She has always feared that men will find her inadequate and unattractive, so she avoids dates with them just like she avoids all other encounters.

Trisha was diagnosed as having social phobia. Supportive and exploratory therapy did not help her, nor did brief contact with Toastmasters, a worldwide speaking skills organization. A psychiatrist started her on behavioral therapy, which helped Trisha identify her faulty and distressing thoughts. But she still feels uptight all day and night. With her doctor's approval, Trisha has started taking kava, which has made her feel even better, especially in situations she avoided in the past. Now Trisha no longer fears blushing in any encounter.

The following list contains typical impairments caused by each anxiety disorder. If you can identify with any of these lists, see a doctor for a thorough evaluation.

Social Phobia

- Avoiding social contact
- Unable to write a check or sign a credit card slip while being watched

- Unable to hold down a job
- Unable to go for an interview
- Unable to urinate in a public restroom
- Avoiding restaurants, cafeterias
- Blushing or profuse sweating in public
- Using alcohol to reduce social anxiety
- Feeling depressed and suicidal
- Unable to stand up for one's self or speak one's mind without great distress
- Failing to achieve full professional potential

Panic Disorder

- Visits to emergency department with acute chest pain, thinking you are dying of a heart attack
- Difficulty driving on busy streets due to fear
- Avoiding elevators, escalators, airplanes
- Avoiding crowded places or places where there's no escape if you have a panic attack
- Unable to go to a PTA meeting or to watch your child perform at a school event
- Social withdrawal and isolation in more severe cases
- Frustration or discomfort associated with persistence of symptoms after many medical evaluations

Generalized Anxiety Disorder

- Irritability, angry spells at family members
- Many visits to doctors for physical problems (headache, chest pain, bowel symptoms, tiredness, muscle stiffness, fear of serious disease without basis)—generally feels doctor has not understood or helped patient
- Worry that your child has not come home on time and has therefore been hurt or killed
- Worry that, if you are late, others will get angry or disapprove of you as a person
- Worry that you have cancer, AIDS, a brain tumor, or the like, based on the slightest little ache or pain

- Exhaustion or, conversely, lots of unproductive nervous energy
- Giving up easily while doing things
- Muscle tension that interferes with sleep and daily activities
- Inability to fall asleep due to incessant worrying, frequently over trivial matters

When Self-Help Isn't Enough

If any of the following are true, we recommend that you see a doctor for evaluation and/or treatment. Do *not* self-administer kava if . . .

- Your symptoms cause you much distress and are interfering with your relationships and at home/work/school.
- Your symptoms are interfering significantly with either your work, family, or social life.
- You have started to use alcohol or drugs to cope.
- You are experiencing depression, a sense of hopelessness, or suicidal ideas.
- Your physical health is not good, and you find it hard to accomplish routine activities and responsibilities.
- You are taking other medication from your doctor, for another medical problem, and are thinking about self-medication with an herbal remedy.
- You have had trouble with abuse of or dependence on other anxiety-reducing medicine or alcohol.
- You suffer from *serious* depression. Although kava may have some antidepressant or mood-elevating effects, at this stage of our knowledge it cannot be recommended on its own for depression. Major depression (see page 40) needs medical attention and probably treatment with an antidepressant drug, St. John's wort, or a specialized form of psychotherapy—as discussed in Chapter 1.
- You are pregnant or planning to conceive. In these circumstances, the use of any form of medication is best avoided unless absolutely necessary. This would include kava. Although there is no evidence that this herb is associated with any damage to the baby, studies have not been done, and it is a general principle not to take medications during pregnancy unless absolutely necessary and on your doctor's recommendation.

- You are already taking other drugs that sedate or impair your alertness (see page 133 for details).
- You are under age 18.

Five Good Reasons to Take Kava

Kava might be a good remedy for you if you fit these descriptions:

- You're experiencing the symptoms of stress but don't have a clinical anxiety disorder.
- You have a clinical anxiety disorder and simply do not want to take more conventional forms of treatment. **Note:** you should discuss this with a doctor.
- You've had troublesome side effects from a variety of different medicines you've tried for anxiety or stress.
- Other medicines have failed to work.
- You are already receiving cognitive-behavioral therapy and wish to add a mild anti-anxiety medicine but do not want to see yet another therapist or doctor.

If I do have an anxiety disorder, can it be cured?

Anxiety disorders are chronic, that is, lasting for several years, and typically follow an undulating course. All treatments (enumerated below) help relieve symptoms, but to our knowledge no one has yet studied whether any form of anti-anxiety treatment can prevent the development of anxiety or cure it permanently. Only about 20 to 25 percent of those treated for anxiety achieve a complete cure. Another 20 percent or so continue to have serious problems controlling their anxiety. The middle group, about 50 to 60 percent, usually gain substantial improvement but still manifest some symptoms.

We have some evidence that relapse is not very common following completion of cognitive-behavioral therapy. In one German study by Volz and Kieser (1997) kava was found to have had a sustained response for up to six months. Those who respond well to prescription anti-anxiety medications usually also get a sustained response over long periods of time. But so far there is no evidence that any treatment or lifestyle change increases the rate of cure.

The exceptions are adjustment disorders with anxious mood and acute stress disorder. In these cases, once the originating stress passes, in the former disorder, or after three or four weeks in the latter disorder, the symptoms often do disappear.

What this boils down to is that treatments for all the anxiety disorders usually need to be long term. The chance of symptoms returning is reasonably high if treatment is stopped; even with continued treatment, there is likely to be some continuation of symptoms, albeit at a lower level than before treatment.

Treatment Options

If your anxiety is mild and infrequent, or if you are having just one or two isolated symptoms, lifestyle changes alone may help you, especially if you can determine that some aspect of your lifestyle may be causing or contributing to your symptoms. Otherwise, treatment choices for anxiety break into three broad groups: psychotherapy, medications, and lifestyle modifications.

Cognitive-behavioral therapy (CBT) can be very effective for all the anxiety disorders. Indeed, it seems to work as well as medication in all but the most severe cases. In many cases CBT is combined with some form of medication, including kava. CBT differs from the more traditional forms of "talk" therapy in that it is highly structured, requiring you to work hard between sessions at a variety of tasks and exercises prescribed by the therapist, usually over a period of weeks or months. To oversimplify, the point of cognitive-behavioral therapy is to give you a new way of thinking, and behaving, that will alleviate your symptoms. In the case of anxiety disorders, this may mean gradually and repeatedly exposing yourself to the people, situations, objects, or events that you fear and have been avoiding.

You could also be asked to keep a daily diary to identify and challenge faulty and distressing beliefs that may underlie your anxiety. Taking such steps can, at first, increase your discomfort. Thus many people discontinue their therapy midway because of the effort and discomfort involved. However, it is worth noting that recent clinical research indicates that CBT may be the best way to erase long-standing fears and phobias, by creating new, positive associations regarding the feared object that are stronger than the old, negative associations.

If you're interested in CBT, consider reading any of the following books: *Anxiety Disorders and Phobias: A Cognitive Perspective*, by Aaron T. Beck et al. (Basic Books, 1990); *Stop Obsessing*, by Edna B. Foa et al. (Bantam Books, 1991); *Don't Panic: Taking Control of Anxiety Attacks*, by Reid Wilson (Harper Perennial, 1996); and *The Hidden Face of Shyness*, by Franklin Schneier and Lawrence Welkowitz (Avon Books, 1996).

Anxiolytic Medications

Half a century ago the main medications prescribed for anxiety were the barbiturates, whose effectiveness came at the cost of addiction, extreme sedation, depression, and danger of overdose. By the 1960s these drugs had been supplanted by the benzodiazepines: Valium (diazepam), Librium (chloradiazepoxide), and Serax (oxazepam). Xanax and Klonopin (clonazepam) have been added more recently. While these drugs had the advantage of working very quickly (often within an hour of administration) and of less commonly producing bothersome side effects, they came with their own negative baggage: the possibility of sedation, unsteadiness, fatigue, or sexual difficulties; a small risk of addiction; and a relatively high risk of physical dependence and withdrawal symptoms. Nor do they have any effect on obsessive–compulsive disorder, posttraumatic stress disorder, or depression.

The latest and most promising generation of psychotropic drugs for treating anxiety is actually the class of antidepressants called the SSRIs (see Chapter 1 for more details on this class of drugs). While these drugs also have side effects, with the exception of Buspar (buspirone), which is not strictly an SSRI but works mainly on serotonin) they seem to be effective in OCD, PTSD, GAD, social phobia, and panic disorder with or without agoraphobia. Buspar seems to be effective only in GAD but is perhaps also useful in reducing alcohol consumption in people who have GAD with alcohol abuse. A newer class of medications currently finding favor in the field is the anticonvulsants, which may work through their effects on GABA or another brain chemical called *glutamate*.

How Kava Can Help with Anxiety

As with other herbal remedies—and, indeed, alternative medical practices in general—Europe is way ahead of the United States in the medicinal use of kava. In Germany, for example, kava is commonly prescribed
for nervous anxiety, stress, insomnia, and restlessness. As one of us
(Connor; see Connor and Vaughan, 1999) reported recently, almost 100
tons of kava are imported into Europe every year, and roughly 350,000
prescriptions for kava are written in Germany alone. Standardized extracts of kavalactones, the active ingredient in kava (see page 95), have
been approved for such uses not only in Germany but also in the United
Kingdom, Switzerland, and Austria. The research studies done on kava's
use for anxiety stack up to a much smaller pile than those for St. John's
wort, ginkgo, and valerian, but the evidence from published trials all
points to kava's effectiveness.

Three double-blind studies conducted in Germany have evaluated
kava and a placebo in patients suffering from anxiety states. The criteria
used to define anxiety states in these studies were rather loose, but they
overlap broadly with the symptoms of GAD, panic disorder/agoraphobia,
and social phobia.

In the first study, Warneke (1991) and his colleagues studied women
with menopause-related symptoms of anxiety and gave either kava at a
dose of 210 mg of kavalactones per day or placebo. Using the Hamilton
Anxiety Scale (see page 113), they observed a significant difference in favor of kava as early as one week into the test and throughout the rest of
treatment. With kava, the overall symptom level had been reduced by
more than 75 percent, whereas with placebo, it was reduced less than 30
percent.

In a second study, by Lehmann and colleagues (1996), 58 patients who
met diagnostic criteria for anxiety disorders received 210 mg of kavalactones per day for four weeks. Again by the end of week 1 there was evidence that kava was more effective than placebo. This difference continued to increase as treatment went on. By the end of four weeks, 52 percent
of the kava group had been judged to respond to treatment, while only 17
percent of the placebo group had responded.

In a third study, Volz and Keiser (1997) gave kava or placebo to 101
patients suffering from anxiety disorders as defined by the third revised edition of the *Diagnostic and Statistical Manual* (DSM-III-R), the standard set
of diagnostic criteria in use at the time. In this study, the effect of kava took

somewhat longer to appear, but by week 8 and continuing thereafter it was superior to placebo on the Hamilton Anxiety Scale. Seventy-five percent of the kava group responded positively, as compared to 51 percent of the placebo group.

Two additional German studies compared one brand of kava, Neuronika, which contains the kavalactone *d,l*-kavain, against anxiety-reducing benzodiazepine drugs (Xanax, Valium, and Klonopin in the United States) and/or bromazepam in anxiety disorders. In one study, Lindenberg and Pitule-Schodel (1990) studied 38 patients with an anxiety disorder diagnosis, and found that kava and oxazepam (less widely used in the United States but a good comparison since it has demonstrated anti-anxiety effects) were equally effective, without producing any troublesome side effects. In the second study, Woelke (1993) gave subjects either kava, oxazepam, or another benzodiazepine drug, bromazepam (which is unavailable in North America). In this study, all patients met diagnostic criteria for anxiety disorder according to the *International Classification of Diseases* (ICD) of the World Health Organization (WHO). All three treatments produced the same effects on anxiety as measured by the Hamilton Anxiety Scale.

One of the problems with these two studies is that they included no placebo control, which means that all they demonstrate is that kava seems to do as well as a standard treatment. They do not show that kava (or benzodiazepine, for that matter) is better than no treatment at all.

None of the studies done so far tell us whether kava would be as good as a benzodiazepine or an antidepressant (which can also work well for anxiety) in more severe cases. Such studies are desperately needed, but as far as we know none are ongoing or planned at this time. We compare the key properties of each major treatment approach in Table 7.

Is kava effective for all the anxiety disorders?

The biggest question that remains about what kava can do for anxiety is whether it is effective in all the individual anxiety disorders. Kava does seem to be helpful for people with symptoms of generalized anxiety disorders (GAD), social phobia, and panic disorder, though a few doctors may resist prescribing any type of medicine for panic disorder on the theory that patients become too dependent on it. We really do not know at this time how useful kava might be for obsessive–compulsive disorder or posttraumatic stress disorder, or for more severe forms of the other disorders.

Table 7. Comparison of Four Different Treatment Approaches
for Anxiety Disorder

	Anxiolytics	Anti-depressants	CBT	Kava
Evidence of efficacy	+++	+++	+++	++
Side effects	++	+++	+	+
Adverse interactions with other medication	+	+	–	?
Relapse after stopping treatment	+++	++	–	?
Ease of treatment for participant	+++	+++	+	+++

Note. +++, strong likelihood; ++, moderate likelihood; +, low likelihood; ?, unknown; –, none/little.

Our clinical experience has demonstrated that kava can be very help-ful in GAD. GAD is a state of heightened worry and tension that the suf-ferer finds hard to control, which is present more than 50 percent of the time for at least six months, and is accompanied by at least three of these symptoms: insomnia, poor concentration, muscle tension, fatigue, irritabil-ity, and tension.

Forty-year-old Martha complained of increasing levels of tension, find-ing it very difficult to control her anxiety, irritability, and physical symp-toms. She had bothersome headaches and muscle tension in her shoulders. She woke up too early, was startled too easily, had to urinate too often, and had lost much of her sexual drive. In short, anxiety seemed to hurt Martha in every facet of her daily life.

We diagnosed her with GAD and prescribed an anticonvulsant drug called Neurontin (gabapentin), which helped Martha feel much more re-laxed for a while but negatively affected her memory and powers of concen-tration. We decided to replace Neurontin with up to 500 mg per day of kava because Martha had read good things about it and we had been using it successfully with other patients.

One of the first benefits Martha noticed was that kava helped her go to sleep and stay asleep, leaving her a lot more refreshed in the morning and thus a lot less irritable and a lot sharper during the day. At last she felt like she was getting done what needed to be done. Martha also found that kava helped her keep her worries out of the bedroom, which increased her desire and her enjoyment of sex with her husband.

Still, Martha's symptoms sometimes came back, so we decided to increase her dose of kava to 1 gram (1,000 mg) per day. Now Martha felt better almost all the time, suffering fewer ups and downs and no side effects. Interestingly, she felt so good about the effect of kava that she recommended it to her husband, who started to take it himself. As a result, he grew less consumed by the worries of running his own business.

Will kava work safely and effectively for the whole course of anxiety?

As we mentioned earlier, only one study Volz and Kieser (1996) so far has evaluated the effects of kava for as long as six months. This study did find it to be effective for this length of time, but clinical anxiety disorders often last much longer, so we need to study whether kava will in fact stay effective throughout the entire course. This issue is of less importance for those who suffer episodic symptoms of stress, though it would also be interesting to know whether taking kava over a long period would prevent such symptoms from returning. Many people who know the damage stress can do would gladly take kava over the long haul, the way many of us take vitamin C to protect ourselves from colds, if they thought it would exert a preventive effect.

Experience in some Australian Aboriginal communities shows that some individuals who take kava at extremely high doses over a period of several years can develop malnutrition, shortness of breath, general ill health, loss of weight, liver damage, and changes in blood cells. These findings are, however, by no means typical or realistic risks for most people who use kava in therapeutic doses on an occasional basis. It is quite likely that the use of kava simply complicated the already poor health of the Australian Aboriginals who had these characteristics.

I've been seeing a doctor for fairly severe anxiety for three years, and I'm tired of constantly taking prescription drugs. Do you think kava might be a good replacement for Buspar?

We do not yet know for sure if kava is likely to help more severe anxiety, but the evidence so far suggests that it can be beneficial in a range of anxiety symptoms from mild to moderately severe. Perhaps, in more severe anxiety, it could still be useful as an adjunct to other forms of therapy like regular medication (but under a doctor's care), behavioral treatments, and/or participation in a support group.

*I have a really important interview next week. Can I take kava
right before it to help me get over the jitters and be at my best?*

Some people do find that kava relaxes and calms them for events that require poise and presence of mind. But not everyone gets the same effects
from kava, so we recommend that you try a test dose ahead of time—possibly right now. Try a dose between 140 and 210 mg of kavalactones. If that
dose doesn't give you a strong enough benefit, you can continue your test,
increasing the dose until you find the best level for you.

Once you know that kava is likely to help put you in the best frame of
mind for your interview, you can take the dose you've arrived at either a
couple of hours beforehand or, if your interview is in the morning, even the
night before.

*I started taking kava a month ago and my social life has
improved so much that I'm now seeing one woman on a regular
basis, and things couldn't be better. I don't want to take this herb
forever, but I'm really afraid that if I stop taking it I'll turn from a
prince into the frog I used to be. Will that happen?*

We generally recommend continuing on a successful medication or herbal
remedy for at least 9 to 12 months in social phobia, especially if it has been
present for several years, as is usually the case. You can taper over a few
weeks when you feel ready, but there is at least a 50 percent chance, if not
more, that your symptoms will return in the first year. You are more likely
to relapse if you have been profoundly shy and avoidant of most people, if
you have a strong family history of anxiety, and if you have had other problems like depression.

*I've been diagnosed as having both generalized anxiety disorder
and social phobia. Can kava help me?*

Many people, like you, suffer from more than one form of anxiety. In a
study we conducted in the North Carolina population (Davidson et al.
1993), we found that there was a greater than threefold chance of having
generalized anxiety if an individual also had social phobia. While 8 percent
of the population without social phobia had experienced generalized anxiety, the rate among those with social phobia was 27 percent. Unfortunately,
until studies are done to test kava not only with each individual disorder

but also with various combinations of these disorders, we won't know whether kava is the best answer, or even a good answer, to comorbidity in anxiety disorders. Since, however, the same drug can often help with both social phobia and generalized anxiety disorder, it certainly makes sense to try kava.

My 75-year-old-mother has always been a worrier, but now that my father is in a nursing home she seems to be getting much worse, never sleeping through the night, having difficulty concentrating, and getting extremely upset over little things as well as big ones. Would it be safe for her to try kava?

Kava can be taken by an adult of any age, although it is generally wise to start with smaller doses and increase gradually if you are above age 65. In fact, these are wise cautions observed in prescribing essentially any prescription drug in the elderly. As people age, they experience changes in drug metabolism and distribution. They also have increased sensitivity to side effects. Note, in fact, that mild transient side effects observed in the average adult can be more problematic in the elderly. For example, unsteadiness can lead to falls, which may result in broken hips. The elderly are also much more likely to experience confusion in response to medications, which can have serious consequences. Older adults are also more likely to have other chronic medical problems and to use other (often multiple) medications that might result in herb–drug interactions (see pages 153–154).

My son is very nervous and seems to fret over his schoolwork and friendships much more than other 10-year-olds. Could we give him kava?

We would caution against giving kava to anyone in this age group until other means have been tried. Before deciding to treat, we believe a comprehensive medical and psychological evaluation is advisable.

One of my friends said kava really helped him lick the blues. Should I try it when I'm feeling depressed?

Whether kava can be used successfully to treat depression is a somewhat fuzzy issue. We would not customarily recommend it for depression since it has not been shown to have any antidepressant effects. But if what you describe more closely fits the profile of mild to moderate stress (see pages 36–43)—which can certainly make you feel dejected—kava may in fact lift your spirits. Although other sources caution against its use in severe depression, we have not seen anyone become depressed while taking kava. If you decide to try kava for symptoms that resemble depression (see pages 101–103 in Chapter 1), make your trial brief. If your symptoms persist or worsen, stop taking kava and see your doctor.

Friends tell me kava has enhanced their sex life. Is there any scientific evidence for this claim?

Some herbs, such as ginkgo (discussed in Chapter 3), can have sexually enhancing effects under certain circumstances. We have no scientific evidence to support the notion that kava has direct aphrodisiac properties, but this claim has certainly been made by some of our patients and in Polynesian lore.

Several of kava's main effects might explain why someone taking it might feel that his or her sex life has been enhanced. First, the increased awareness of sensations that people report with kava may extend to increased awareness and enjoyment of sexual pleasure. Second, and a more plausible possibility, is that by reducing symptoms of stress or preoccupation with its causes, kava can put you in a better physical and mental state to be able to enjoy intimacy and sexual pleasure. Although this aspect of kava has not been reported in any of the clinical studies, it is quite reasonable to expect such an indirect benefit, as would be the case with any effective treatment for stress or anxiety.

I noticed that kava was included with the other remedies for insomnia at my health food store. Will it work as well as the other herbs used for sleeplessness?

Sleeplessness can be caused by all kinds of factors, both biological and environmental, so most people find that they have to experiment to identify the best possible sleeping aid among the various herbs that might help. Valerian is considered primarily a remedy for insomnia; we discuss it in Chapter 4. If insomnia is your main problem and it's chronic, you might want to try valerian first, after reading Chapter 4. But if what seems to keep you awake are symptoms of anxiety—for example, you start worrying before bedtime and can't quiet your mind, you get tense and have a hard time relaxing physically, or the fight-or-flight feeling of panic keeps you wide awake—kava might be an especially good choice.

Kava can improve insomnia and does not seem to produce any morning-after hangover effects. Lebot et al. (1997) have suggested a dose of 500 to 800 mg of kavalactones for sleep enhancement, although we have noted good results at lower doses such as 140 to 210 mg, taken two or three hours before bedtime. Another study found that kava increased the amount of restorative slow-wave sleep, without any evidence of symptom rebound on stopping it (Connor and Vaughan, 1999, pp. 99–100).

A friend told me she has thrown away her aspirin and ibuprofen and now uses only kava instead. Does the herb really work the same way as over-the-counter painkillers?

Many people have reported that pain can be lessened on kava. Experiments have also shown this to be true, but so far the mechanism has not been worked out. For mild pain from muscle tension to joint pain or headache, kava may be helpful. It is possible that the historical use of kava for urinary tract infections relates to its ability to reduce the burning sensations on urination that often accompany a bladder infection. However, its use for this indication is now only of historical interest.

Kava may have anti-inflammatory effects, operating as a type of "ibuprofen." Kava can inhibit cyclo-oxygenase and thromboxane, enzymes that promote the formation of prostaglandin E2 and thromboxane E2, both of which mediate the inflammatory response. To what extent these actions of kava are therapeutically significant is unknown at present.

Kava is by no means a narcotic, as some sources have reported. But most anxiolytics are sedative at higher doses, and kava probably works on a very similar mechanism. Its anxiety-reducing powers have shown it is a tranquillizer. These types of effects may have misled some people to believe that kava falls among more powerful drugs like narcotics.

❦ HOW KAVA WORKS

The Kava Plant

James Cook named it *Piper methysticum*, or "intoxicating pepper," for the effects he observed among the Polynesians who introduced it to him. The

Polynesians called it *kava*, for "bitter," after the distinctly unpleasant taste that the root or its extract leaves in the mouth. Of the large number of species contained in the *Piper* genus, kava is one of the few with medicinal properties. Most of us are familiar with *Piper nigram*, which gives us black and white peppers. You may have heard of *Piper betle*, which contains a stimulant, arecoline, and is chewed for its mind-altering effects throughout much of Southeast Asia.

Kava is a shrub found only in the South Pacific islands. It is cultivated in a manner comparable to sugarcane. Cut kava stalks are laid in mud trenches until they sprout. After sprouting, the stalks are planted in shallow trenches, where they take approximately six or seven years to reach maturity and their full height of up to 10 feet. The mature plant contains relatively few heart-shaped leaves that are four to 10 inches long.

When the plant is mature, the kava roots, or rhizomes, are ready for harvesting. It is from these roots that the active medicine is extracted. The root itself may be sold whole, cut, powdered, or dried. Customarily, each kava plantation remains in the same family through successive generations.

Different varieties of kava exist in Hawaii, the Marquesas Islands, Fiji, Samoa, and New Guinea. In Vanuatu, which supplies a large amount of the kava consumed in the United States, there are 72 different varieties of kava. The different varieties can be recognized by varying spaces between stem joints in the plant, color of stems, quality of roots, and intensity of leaf color. While all of the varieties of kava can be expected to have some degree of medicinal and psychoactive effects, the exact amount of kava-lactones (also called *kavapyrones*), which contain the active medicinal compound, may vary. This means differences in the intensity and quality of the psychological effect may be apparent to some individuals. Pacific islanders were apparently well acquainted with these distinctions, assigning different varieties different uses—for example, some were reserved for chiefs in religious ceremonies and others were used by the general population for everyday purposes.

As we mentioned earlier in the chapter, German biochemical researchers isolated the 15 kavalactones in kava around the turn of the century. But it wasn't until the middle of the century that Professor Hans Myer, at the Freiburg University Institute of Pharmacology, analyzed the activities of the kavalactones. Through animal studies, he found that six of them—kavain, dihydrokavain, methysticin, dihydromethysticin, yangonin, and desmethoxy-yangonin—exhibited sedative, anti-anxiety, pain-relieving, muscle-relaxing, and anticonvulsant effects. These findings have since largely been borne out in studies using human subjects.

Kava and the Brain

The human brain is wired to help us interpret incoming information from our environment, to make sense of or appraise it, and then to produce some form of appropriate response. Anything that could be frightening activates fear signals in a part of the brain called the *limbic system*, whose job it is to emotionally evaluate incoming impressions and then produce a response of either fight or flight. In anxiety, the response is normally one of flight—people with anxiety disorders typically avoid feared situations.

Although we do not understand the mechanisms of kava's effects very well, studies have shown that kava affects an almond-shaped organism in the limbic system called the *amygdala*, reducing the intensity of fear responses. Kava's anxiolytic and sedative effects may relate to receptor activity of GABA, not only in the amygdala but also in the hippocampus and medulla oblongata regions of the brain. Serotonin and glutamate may also be involved. Specifically, kava seems to enhance the effect of serotonin and GABA, which can both result in lowered anxiety, while reducing the effect of glutamate, a chemical that itself can cause increased arousal and distress. Although what we know comes from studies of anxiety, it's likely that kava's actions work neurologically pretty much the same way in stress.

Kava's muscle-relaxing and anticonvulsant effects may be due to inhibition of voltage-dependent sodium channels in muscles and the brain. Its pain-relieving effects may be due to the inhibition of cyclo-oxygenase and thromboxane, enzymes involved in the production of inflammation-causing chemicals (prostaglandin and thromboxane), as we noted earlier.

How Safe Is Kava?

As with all the herbal remedies considered "dietary supplements" by the FDA, kava has not passed the rigorous safety tests required of prescription or even over-the-counter drugs. Nor has it undergone scientific testing as extensively as St. John's wort. Collectively, the clinical, anecdotal, and research evidence indicates that kava is comparatively safe, but not necessarily in all circumstances, at all doses, for all individuals. We simply don't know enough yet about how kava works under all possible conditions to give it an all-clear for safety. The myth that so-called natural remedies like herbs are inherently safe is just that—a myth. Where any psychoactive substance is concerned, caution is required.

The truth is that any sedating substance can be dangerous if its effects are exaggerated. We know of one patient who took kava and the prescription anxiolytic Xanax and was admitted to the emergency room after going into a coma. We don't know the details of this case, but it served as a warning to make us be on the alert in our own clinical practice for potential interaction problems between kava and other sedatives or tranquilizers. It's a fact that kava can increase the sedative properties of a number of tranquilizing medications such as anticonvulsants, benzodiazepines (e.g., Xanax), and certain antidepressants. Until we have more data informing us of the threshold for dangerous interactions and potentiations, we intend to err on the side of overcaution.

How Kava Works Compared to Prescription Anxiolytics

There are a number of important differences between kava and the very widely used benzodiazepines drugs (see Table 8). Many of the prescription drugs used to treat anxiety can cause dependence, and they also have at least a slightly greater potential for causing other negative side effects.

Table 8 indicates kava may be safer to use than the benzodiazepines. Note, however, that the chart assumes fairly small doses of kava. At higher doses, kava–alcohol interaction could very well be a problem. We'll discuss that topic on pages 133–134, but first let's see how kava stacks up in terms of side effects.

What Side Effects to Expect from Kava

Very few side effects were noted in the clinical studies of kava described earlier in this chapter. In the biggest study, which evaluated approximately 50 subjects on kava and 50 on placebo, only five of the kava patients expe-

Table 8. Kava versus Benzodiazepines

Effect	Kava	Benzodiazepine drugs
Increased alertness	Yes	No
Increased effects of alcohol	No	Yes
Potential to increase aggression	No	Sometimes

rienced a total of six side effects, in four of which the doctor did not think that the treatment had any relation to the side effect. In the placebo group, nine patients reported 15 mild side effects, which tells us that it is not always the drug that should be blamed when a "side effect" develops. Nonetheless, from our own clinical use of kava, we have observed periodic side effects, including stomach discomfort, headache, and a sense of being "washed out" or exhausted. Only at excessively high doses does kava predictably produce untoward or unpleasant side effects, including extreme tiredness, profound relaxation, "flaccidity" (or looseness of the muscles), and unsteadiness. At this point it might appear that the kava drinker appears inebriated and will often fall asleep.

Benzodiazepine drugs can impair performance, reduce alertness, and interfere with memory. In studies that compared kava with oxazepam, kava actually was found to enhance concentration, increase alertness, and increase the rate at which new words were recognized. All of the measures were impaired to some degree by oxazepam. So not only is kava apparently superior to oxazepam (and presumably other benzodiazepine drugs) on these measures, but it almost certainly affects the brain in a different way in terms of its anxiety-reducing effects. In a study that looked at the interaction between kava and the effects of alcohol in healthy volunteers, no increased effect of alcohol was observed, whereas with oxazepam the effect of alcohol was increased (Münte et al., 1993). Remember, though, that the test used relatively small doses of kava.

Sometimes people who take higher doses of kava for a long time develop a scaly, fishlike quality to their skin. This condition, called *kava dermopathy*, is unlikely to be a problem for people who use the drug in moderation or on an occasional basis. It has been noted for the most part in Australia among Aboriginals who have developed extremely high use patterns of kava and who are often malnourished. It is therefore unclear what causes kava dermopathy, but it should certainly be considered as a potential side effect for heavy users. Sometimes the skin can also turn a faint yellowish color. These problems generally disappear when kava is stopped.

If you have had a history of skin problems and are considering using kava, we would recommend that you consult a dermatologist.

Kava and Alcohol

Does kava increase the effects of alcohol or does alcohol increase the effects of kava? These are legitimate questions, because other anxiety-reducing drugs, such as the benzodiazepines, do increase the effects of alcohol, creating a potential hazard for someone who is not expecting to be impaired. A study by Herberg (1993) in Germany explored whether kava and alcohol interacted with each other. Interestingly, Herberg found that kava did not potentiate the effects of alcohol in healthy male and female volunteers and, in fact, concentration was enhanced in subjects who received alcohol and kava, as compared to alcohol and placebo. While we would not therefore suggest that you go out and take the two together to boost your powers of concentration, we think the results suggest that some of the mental impairment that alcohol can cause is lessened by kava.

Nonetheless, we would caution you against mixing the two, again because not enough data have come in. At doses higher than the usual therapeutic doses described in this book we don't know how alcohol will interact with kava. And even at lower doses of kava, a large amount of alcohol could well cause a problem.

If you insist on taking this chance, two words of advice are in order: (1) exercise moderation in the amounts you take of both substances and (2) do not drive while under their influence. Interestingly, even without alcohol, kava can cause problematic intoxication if enough is taken. In Utah, a driver who was intoxicated after taking very high doses of kava was recently given a citation for driving under the influence, setting a precedent that should serve as fair warning for anyone assuming that kava is benign just because it is "natural."

Is Kava Addictive?

Drugs and chemicals that reduce anxiety and have a general calming effect have the potential to be abused and to result in physical dependence. This is well known with the older anxiety-reducing drugs such as the barbiturates, which have almost entirely fallen out of use. Drugs like the benzodiazepines (Xanax, Valium, Klonopin) can lead to physical dependence in a certain number of people. Thus it is always prudent to stop these drugs slowly to avoid the distressing withdrawal symptoms that may develop after sudden discontinuation.

On the basis of clinical tradition, kava is not believed to be likely to cause physical dependence or withdrawal symptoms, but it cannot yet be entirely exonerated. A number of reports from Australian Aboriginal societies have suggested that people can become dependent on kava, particularly after taking very high doses for a long time. There is also a report from New Zealand suggesting that kava can be given to help wean people off benzodiazepine drugs like Xanax and to produce less discomfort. On the one hand, this is good news, but on the other hand, it suggests that some of the physical-dependence-producing effects of the benzodiazepines may also be found with kava in a milder form, which may be why kava helps to blunt the symptoms. Similarly, the fact that kava, like the benzodiazepines and barbiturates, acts quickly is reason to be concerned about its potential to be addictive.

If you have had problems with addiction or drug dependence, or find it difficult to control your intake of alcohol, kava may not be for you. On the other hand, it may still be a better choice than some other treatments to help reduce your tension and stress. You should definitely consult with your doctor about this.

❧ HOW TO USE KAVA

When British explorer Captain James Cook sailed through the Pacific during the late 18th century, he was accompanied by naturalist Georg Forster, who returned to Europe with descriptions of the process by which kava was prepared on the island of Fiji. First the root was cut into small pieces, then the pieces were chewed and mixed with coconut milk, then the mixture was drunk from a communal bowl.

Although kava is still often prepared via the ancient ceremonial method in the Pacific islands, in the West it's available in jars and bottles, as capsules, tinctures, and topical preparations, like any other dietary supplement or over-the-counter medicine. We have yet to determine what the best form and dosage are for everyone, so if you plan to try kava, be ready to try different doses within the accepted range.

Dosage

Clinical studies have evaluated doses of 210 mg of kavalactones per day, so that has become the standard recommended daily dose. This amount may often be sufficient for coping with symptoms of stress or anxiety, but sometimes you will find it necessary to increase the dose if you have not responded sufficiently. In our practice, we have given doses more than twice as high, at 500 mg or so of kavalactones. Sometimes we have found this to make a difference, without any problematic side effects.

For mild stress, even 70 mg of kavalactones might be enough. Try this dose and see. For mild to moderate anxiety, we suggest you start with 140 mg per day, then increase your daily dose to 210 mg per day after a week if you're not satisfied with the effect you're getting. You might increase the dose to 280 mg two or three weeks later if you have had no side effects and still feel you haven't improved. Higher doses are fine too, but beyond a dosage of 280 mg you should consider taking kava under medical supervision if you plan to take it for more than two months. Given the basic safety of kava and the lack of side effects, it may be reasonable to try doses up to at least double the usual dose—420 mg of kavalactones or six capsules of 70 mg of kavalactones per day—but again, we advise you to do so only under professional supervision.

Most available brands of kava are standardized to contain a certain amount of kavalactones or kavapyrones, the active ingredient. The bottle label should state the total milligram dose in each capsule (e.g., "384 mg of concentrated kava root"), standardized to a certain percentage of kavalactones (e.g., 55 percent). A capsule containing 384 mg of concentrated kava root, standardized to 55 percent kavalactones, would give you a daily dose of about 210 mg of kavalactones in one capsule. A capsule that contained 128 mg of concentrated kava root extract, standardized to 55 percent of kavalactones, would give you 70 mg of kavalactones, which would mean you would need to take three capsules to get a 210-mg daily dose. The most important thing is to make sure that this kind of information is included on the label of the brand you buy. If it is not included, do not buy or use that brand.

Excessive doses, as used in some of the Australian Aboriginal communities, would be in the grams-per-day range, which means at least 10 times the dose used in regular practice.

I took one capsule of kava and felt really spacy and sort of high. What does that mean?

It may mean that the effect that kava provides just isn't for you. But it might also mean that you've taken more than you need to alleviate stress or anxiety. Check the label and see how much kavalactone was in that one capsule. If it was more than 70 mg, it might be more than you need. If you're interested enough to try again, find another brand that contains less kavalactone per capsule, or buy the kava in another form that will allow you to take a smaller dose.

How and When to Take Kava

If you're taking kava for stress or anxiety, you can take it once or twice a day. Some of our patients have found that taking kava on an empty stomach causes stomach discomfort, so we recommend taking it with food.

For insomnia, take the full day's dose of kava at night, a couple of hours before bedtime. If you find yourself needing kava every night for several weeks, we suggest you consult a doctor about long-term use for insomnia. If you suffer from depression, kava may serve you well as a sleep aid, as long as you are also taking an antidepressant.

About 280 mg of kavalactones has really eased my constant worrying and nervous tension, but it means remembering to take four capsules a day. Can I just take them all at once?

You can try cutting down to one or two doses, depending on what works best for you. For anxiety control (as opposed to sleep), taking 140 mg twice a day is generally better than taking 280 mg all at once. We have no data at this time on how long kava stays in the bloodstream, so personal experimentation is still the best way to determine how best to spread out your total daily dose.

How Kava Is Sold

Kava is available in pill, capsule, liquid, tea, and spray forms. Perhaps because tablets and capsules camouflage most of kava's inherently bitter taste, these forms seem to be the most popular. Whatever form you choose, be sure you know if the content of the kava has been standardized. The usual amount of active kavalactones ranges from 30 to 70 percent according to brand. Look to see if the kava comes from root extract, since the most medicinally active part of the plant is the root. If extracts have been added from other parts of the plant, like the stem or leaves, the overall effectiveness of the kava may be undermined.

Kava teas, often found in health food stores and some grocery stores, are also quite popular. In general, herbal teas are much less potent than their counterpart tablet or tincture forms. Teas dissolve in water, which usually does not produce as potent a medicine as tinctures, which dissolve in alcohol. However, teas probably do help mild insomnia and also probably do promote some increase in sociability.

Many people believe that hot kava tea has a more relaxing effect than cold tea. Pour hot boiling water over two spoons of powdered kava or ground kava root, and allow the resulting tea to brew for about 10 or 15 minutes. Strain it through filter paper and then drink it.

Tinctures of kava are powder forms of medicine dissolved in alcohol. The proportions of kava to alcohol in a tincture will vary according to brand. It is not always easy to tell from the bottle what these proportions are. In any event, the percentage of alcohol is likely to be quite high in most tinctures. We've already cautioned you against using kava if you have an alcohol problem; obviously, if you still want to try kava to treat your anxiety, you should at least avoid these tinctures forms.

Kava tinctures are ingested via a dropper. They may produce a numbness in the mouth shortly after applying the liquid. This numbness may be taken as a sign that the quality of the brand is good. Because a medicine that is absorbed sublingually (through the tongue) does not undergo absorption through the gut or break down in the liver, it acts more quickly. Thus a tincture might be the best choice for you if your principal need for kava is to relieve stage fright before some stressful event. Tinctures are usually more expensive than pills and capsules, but many people think the cost differential is justified because they believe the tinctures are not only quicker acting but more potent. This claim has not been proven scientifically.

Kava is also available in spray form. One of the apparent advantages of a spray is that it may not have the bitter quality of the tinctures or teas. Unfortunately, the lack of bitterness in some sprays may be due to the low dose of kava they contain. This means, of course, that what you gain in taste you lose in effectiveness.

When I take a capsule or even a tincture, it takes at least a couple of hours for me to feel any increased relaxation. So what's the point of kava bars if you're not going to feel the effect until after you've left?

The kava served in kava bars is prepared in a manner more like that practiced in the South Pacific. The root is macerated and prepared to be consumed as a beverage. In its unprocessed form "bar" kava is often taken in larger quantities, which may explain quicker onset and greater possible effect. In contrast, the preparations available in retail stores are processed differently, through an elaborate manufacturing procedure, which generally leads to an extract form of the product that behaves a bit differently.

Does Brand Matter?

As we have said regarding other herbal products, choosing a brand is not easy, because we do not always have the information we need to make an informed decision. Our best advice is to make sure that the label states whether the product is standardized—but keep in mind that this means only that we know how much of the product contains active kavalactones. A higher percentage of kavalactones does not necessarily mean better effectiveness. Nor does higher cost guarantee better quality. Also be sure that the label includes a lot number, an expiration date, and a manufacturer's name and address.

An informal survey we did of 14 different kava brands, taken from three different stores, produced a confusing picture (see Table 9). Eleven different dose strengths (in terms of milligrams of kavalactone per pill) were available, and one brand gave no indication of dose. Of the eleven different doses, five gave the dose as actual percentage of kavalactones (the active ingredient of kava, or "the part that counts," if you like). In the other cases, the dose given reflected the entire amount of kava, with the standardized percentage of kavalactones provided, which would mean that you have to do some quick math to figure out how much of the actual dose (usually 30 percent) was kavalactones.

Four brands were not standardized, meaning that you could not tell the quantity of kavalactones.

Dosing directions were quite variable, ranging from one per day up to six per day. Nine brands recommended taking kava "as needed," while the other five recommended regular daily doses of up to three per day. In one case, the recommended dose was only 60 mg of kavalactones per day; at the other end of the spectrum one brand recommended 250 mg of kavalactones per day.

In three cases, kava was sold as part of a combination in which hops, schizandra, and chamomile were also present.

The daily cost for a dose of 250 mg of kavalactones or so ranged from $0.60 to $2.40. If you were interested in purchasing the least expensive form of kava from our surveyed brands, it could be obtained for $0.24/day, but since no dose was given, you would have no idea how much kava you were taking. You clearly need to select your brand based on other things than price alone.

Expiration dates were given for only eight brands.

So, if you are thinking about buying kava, look for the dose of

Table 9. Retail Survey of Kava Brands (November 1998)

Brand	Dose/pill	Pills/day	Standardized	Other ingredients	Expiration date	Cost/day[a]
A	425 mg TK	1–3 once daily as needed	No	No	Yes	$0.11–0.33
B	250 mg TK	1 three times a day as needed	30% KL	Yes (3)	Yes	$0.72
C	200 mg TK	1–3 times as needed	30% KL	No	Yes	$0.15–0.45
D	425 mg TK	3 times as needed	No	No	Yes	$0.24
E	460 mg TK	1–4 daily	30% KL	Yes (4)	Yes	$0.15–0.60
F	450 mg TK	2–6 daily	No	No	Yes	$0.10–0.30
G	Not given	15–20 drops three times as needed	No	No	Yes	?
H	60 mg KL	1 three times as needed	30% KL	No	No	$0.99
I	150 mg KL	1–2 once daily	30% KL	No	No	$0.52–1.04
J	75 mg KL	1–3 times as needed	30% KL	No	No	$0.31–0.93
K	200 mg TK	2 twice daily	30% KL	Yes (4)	No	$0.66
L	70 mg KL	1 twice or three times as needed	55% KL	No	Yes	$0.25–0.75
M	10 mg KL	4–6 per day as needed	2–5% KL	No	Yes	$0.20–0.60
N	150 mg TK	1–3 once daily	30% KL	No	No	$0.27–081

Note. TK, total kava dose; KL, kavalactones.
[a]Cost computed based upon dose directions on the bottle.

kavalactones, decide if you want a combination product, make sure there is an expiration date, and remember that for anxiety or sleep you will probably need at least 150 mg of kavalactones, so the recommended dose on the label may not be adequate.

A Few Precautions

Can kava be taken along with other medications for anxiety?

One of our patients who did well on kava was 50-year-old Kurt, whom we had treated for generalized anxiety disorder in a clinical drug trial. Although he responded quite well to the treatment, he felt that he had not made a fully adequate response. He would have periods in the week when he was increasingly tense and worried. During the periods he would pull hairs out of his head as a way of relieving his tension. He was bothered by this behavior, and we decided to treat him with kava. We raised his dose to 500 mg per day. He found within a few weeks that his hair pulling had stopped and that he was a lot less tense and worried. If he took kava on an empty stomach, he would become rather drowsy, so we recommended that he take it with meals; this took care of the problem. Kurt continued to take the Celexa (citalopram) that we had prescribed earlier. On the combination of Celexa and kava he felt that he was doing a lot better.

While Kurt did fine on the combination of a prescription anti-anxiety drug and kava, caution is always required in combining the two. Any drug that causes sleepiness or impairs alertness should be combined with kava only under a doctor's supervision. Examples of such drugs would be sedating antihistamines like Vistaril (hydroxyzine) and Benadryl; tricyclic antidepressants like Elavil (amitriptyline), Sinequan (doxepin), and Tofranil (imipramine); other antidepressants like Desyrel (trazodone), Serzone (nefazodone), and Remeron (mirtazapine); anxiolytics such as the benzodiazepines Xanax, Valium, Klonopin, and Ativan; and alcohol. At high enough doses, kava itself can also have a sedating or alertness-impairing effect.

Can I drive a car or operate machinery if I am taking kava?

As when taking any drug that has sedating effects, you need to be very careful. While kava at the therapeutic dose (210 to 280 mg per day of kavalactones) is not particularly sedating, some individuals may have unusually sensitive responses. Certainly, when you begin to take kava for the first time, you should be very careful not to drive or operate potentially dangerous machinery until you have satisfied yourself that the herb is not affecting you adversely.

*Does kava interact negatively with food or
over-the-counter medicines?*

No such interactions have been documented at this time.

Evaluating Kava's Effectiveness for You

Some of kava's effects—sleepiness, muscle relaxation, tranquility—may be noticeable within just a few hours after taking it. But for the full spectrum of symptoms that come with anxiety disorders, kava usually starts working anywhere between one and four weeks after you take your first dose. Its full benefits may take four to eight weeks to become obvious. For milder stress symptoms, it is likely that kava will help you within a few days, perhaps because there is less "work" to be done by the medicine as compared to the more severe symptoms of an anxiety disorder.

Obviously, if you do not take a high enough dose, kava may never help you. For most people 210 mg of kavalactones will be sufficient, but in some cases the dose may need to be higher. See the procedure for raising your dosage as needed discussed on pages 135–136.

Kava seems to work best for generalized anxiety disorder symptoms. At the moment, there is no good evidence for its benefits in panic disorder, severe social phobia, obsessive–compulsive disorder, or posttraumatic stress disorder. While it is not unreasonable to consider trying kava for these conditions, if it is not helpful, then the best thing would be to try a more proven treatment such as CBT, a benzodiazepine, or an antidepressant drug.

*I'm tired of the side effects of my prescription drug, but my doctor
doesn't ordinarily prescribe kava. How can I convince him to let
me try it instead?*

It is our experience that very few prescribing physicians are aware of kava, although many know something about St. John's wort. While kava still remains somewhat in the shadows, it is actually beginning to emerge into full daylight. As a result, it is quite possible that your doctor will not realize when kava can be used, how it should be used, its safety versus its potential for side effects, and so on. If you are interested in receiving kava from your doctor, you should take some literature to show him at your next visit. A helpful review on kava appeared in *Herbclip*, the abstracting service provided by the American Botanical Council. Some articles from *Herbclip* may be available via its website: www.softlineweb.com/althealth.htm. This useful database of journals in the literature may be able to provide you with full-text articles.

My generalized anxiety has really gotten better thanks to 280 mg of kavalactones every day for the last six months. But now I'm finding that the same dosage doesn't seem to do the trick. What's wrong?

With anxiety, symptoms can often be aggravated by certain substances like caffeine or alcohol, withdrawal from alcohol, and even certain medicines like nasal decongestants (e.g., Sudafed). If any of these are part of your life, they could be triggering your symptoms. To find out, do a little test: simply observe whether there is any association between taking any of these substances and the worsening of your symptoms. You should also mention this problem to your doctor.

Sometimes kava simply loses its effect. Our experience has been that it is better in that case to switch to some other medication than to raise the dose.

How do I know when it's safe to stop taking kava for anxiety?

As with depression, just because your symptoms have gone away does not mean that you should stop taking your medicine! If you decide that this is what you want to do, make sure that you discuss it with your doctor. If you have been self-prescribing, and have remained well for some time, perhaps you could think about stopping treatment. The following would be the best circumstances for doing so:

- Excellent control or symptoms that have disappeared
- Your life is relatively stable and stress-free.

- You have learned skills to cope with stress and anxiety.
- You have decided that it is time to stop taking medicine but not simply in response to some pressures from a magazine, well-meaning friends and relatives, or a therapist who is uncomfortable with the idea of your taking medicine, including herbal remedies.

Many sources also recommend not taking kava for more than three months at a stretch. While one study has shown no ill effects from taking kava for six months, more evidence is needed to make a firm conclusion regarding effectiveness, much less safety, over the long term. We think taking a "medication holiday" after three months is a prudent move for most people who suffer from stress reactions. For anxiety disorders, the issue is a bit more complicated. As a rule, because these conditions are chronic, most doctors recommend staying on your medicine for at least a year—if not longer. So by these principles you would want to stay on kava for as long, presuming it kept working. On the other hand, you should know that data on effectiveness and safety for such a long time simply does not exist, so be sure to discuss this problem with your doctor.

Do I need to taper off kava to stop taking it?

We don't consider tapering necessary for anyone who takes kava on an occasional basis. But if you have been using it every day for any period of time, it is best to taper off. If you've been on kava for three months or less, taper over one week at most. If you've been taking kava for three to 12 months, taper over one to two weeks. If you've been taking it for more than 12 months, taper over two to six weeks. Should you experience any difficulties, such as marked insomnia, nervousness, or other withdrawal-like symptoms, be sure to contact your doctor.

What Lies Ahead?

There are several exciting directions in which kava research might go in the years ahead. We hope, for example, that it will be possible to find out:

- If kava really does improve the daily lives of the many people who experience troublesome stress
- If it can be taken safely and effectively for months or even years

- If it helps all of the anxiety disorders
- Whether there is any real risk of dependency and withdrawal symptoms with regular doses of the herb
- If it could become a safer but equally effective alternative for standard treatment
- If other uses can be established, such as in the treatment of chronic pain.

ESSENTIAL FACTS ABOUT KAVA	
Main Use	Anxiolytic (anti-anxiety treatment), stress relief
Other Reported Uses	Muscle relaxant, sedative/tranquilizer and sleep aid, antidepressant, urinary antiseptic, pain relief, anticonvulsant
When Not to Use This Herb	During pregnancy, when trying to conceive, or breastfeeding; use with caution if under 18 or with alcohol. If taking prescription sedatives, use only under a doctor's supervision.
Side Effects	Stomach discomfort, headache, a sense of being "washed out" or exhausted, "flaccidity" (or looseness of the muscles), unsteadiness, kava dermopathy
When to Expect Positive Effects	Within hours for tension, sleep, muscle relaxation; within two to eight weeks for chronic anxiety
Common Preparation Forms	Pill, capsule, liquid, tea, tincture, spray
Average Effective Daily Dosage	70 to 280 mg of kavalactones (most brands contain concentrated kava root standardized to anywhere from 30 to 70 percent kavalactones; a capsule containing 240 mg of concentrated kava root, standardized to 30 percent, would provide 70 mg of kavalactones), usually taken in divided doses one or two times a day

3

Ginkgo

Fountain of Youth and Vitality

If youth is a fault, it is one which is soon corrected.
—JOHANN WOLFGANG VON GOETHE,
Maxims and Aphorisms

Does the fountain of youth spring from the earth's oldest tree? *Ginkgo biloba*, a plant so ancient that Charles Darwin called it a "living fossil," may be the answer to the baby boomers' hope for a life that is not only longer but also better. Mental sharpness is a hot commodity in today's competitive world, and ginkgo has shown distinct promise for fighting the memory loss and other cognitive problems that accompany age. Even better, it seems to do so safely and inexpensively.

Yet the most intriguing aspect of this ancient herbal remedy may be that its capacity to improve memory and slow the natural mental toll of aging is only the tip of its medicinal iceberg. Study of the mechanisms behind ginkgo's felicitous effect on memory and other cognitive functions reveals that it may also improve the health of blood vessels, alleviate problems with equilibrium and balance, promote the vitality of skin, slow hearing loss, end ringing in the ears, and cure some forms of sexual dysfunction, as well as reduce the damaging effects of radiation and ameliorate altitude sickness.

A persuasive amount of research already attests to ginkgo's potential in all these areas. We believe that future data will probably reinforce ginkgo's promising appeal. As with the other herbs discussed in this book, an important research goal is to perform studies using standards similar to those used by the pharmaceutical industry when it tries to get FDA approval for new drugs. While no details are available at this time, we know the U.S. government, through the National Institutes of Health (NIH), is planning to sponsor a large, controlled, multicenter study of ginkgo in dementia, which is certainly a step in the right direction.

Interestingly, compared to the other herbs discussed in this book, ginkgo seems to be relatively untouched by controversy. The question that needs to be answered for ginkgo may not be "Are the claims made for this herb accurate?" but "Have we taken full advantage of this primeval gift of nature?"

WHAT GINKGO DOES

Over the last century advances in medicine have had a profound effect on life expectancy. People are living longer than ever before. Take 80-year-old Mary, for example. Thanks to good genes (both her grandparents and her parents lived into their eighties), regular activity and exercise, attention to her diet and to stress reduction, Mary is watching her great-grandchildren grow up, keeping up with contemporary fiction, and still volunteering at potluck suppers at her church. Life expectancy for women since she was born has increased from the mid-fifties to around 80, and Mary looks like a promising candidate for another decade of life.

Then there's Frank, also 80, but bound to a wheelchair by a stroke, limited to a soft diet, and unable to read anything but large-print publications. Increasingly confused and forgetful, he has been moved to a nursing home where he will get the round-the-clock supervision and assistance he is beginning to need. The specter of a life like Frank's has become a driving force in the baby boomers' quest to offset and postpone the decline associated with the aging process. The post–World War II generations are determined to keep their bodies fit through good diet and regular exercise, to stave off disease and disability by taking advantage of all the preventive and curative measures that modern medicine offers, and, last but hardly least, to retain all their faculties as long as possible by finding ways to head off the decline in cognitive function that often accompanies old age.

Ginkgo biloba may fill this last niche. (It may contribute to the first two goals as well; more on that later.) Ginkgo has demonstrated positive effects on a number of changes associated with aging. Ginkgo improves blood flow and enhances the integrity of blood vessels. Studies have shown that in the brain, these changes can make people mentally sharper, whether they are already suffering the effects of aging or not. People who have benefited from ginkgo report becoming more alert and attentive, finding it easier to remember all kinds of things—though it's only with time (weeks and months) that these changes become noticeable enough to describe. In other parts of the body, too, ginkgo has been shown to improve conditions associated with poor circulation, such as lightheadedness, dizziness, ringing in the ears, numbness in fingers and toes, and leg pain experienced when walking. Recent research has also shown that ginkgo may have promise for counteracting a troublesome side effect of the widely used newer antidepressants, the SSRIs—namely, problems with sexual arousal and orgasm.

It all sounds too good to be a true: an herbal remedy that seems to be helpful for a variety of ills and may well have preventive or prophylactic effects, that is well tolerated, and that appears to be very safe. While there is substantial evidence already that these claims may be valid, there are dubious exaggerations as well: that ginkgo prevents or cures Alzheimer's disease, that it works for everyone, and that it works for all memory problems. When we gain a better understanding of the various mechanisms of action (how it works), learn more about ginkgo's known clinical applications through properly controlled and well-designed clinical studies, explore new possible applications, and study safety in specific circumstances, we will have a better sense of whether ginkgo can truly be called nature's "fountain of youth."

A Little Ancient History

The ginkgo tree is an ancient plant; indeed, it is the oldest existing tree species, having coexisted with dinosaurs over 200 million years ago. It flourished around the globe until, along with many other plant and animal species, it fell victim to the ravages of the Ice Age. Unlike many other species, however, the ginkgo tree survived the Ice Age, although its growth was limited to parts of eastern Asia in what is now China. Today, thanks to man's intervention, the ginkgo tree flourishes widely once again, growing throughout North America, Europe, and east Asia.

Ginkgo biloba is today the only remaining representative of the Ginkgoaceae family. The ginkgo tree is a *dioecious* species, which means that it has male and female variants. It grows to an average height of 125 feet and lives to the ripe old age of 1,000. The trees do not flower until they are mature, after 20 to 30 years. The male species blossoms in the spring, while adult female trees produce a grayish plumlike fruit that matures and falls in the late autumn months. The fruit pulp has a characteristic foul odor. Ginkgo leaves are particularly unusual for dioecious trees: they have a distinctive bilobed fernlike shape.

Ginkgo biloba is truly nature's resilient wonder. Ginkgo has demonstrated resistance to temperature extremes, insects, microorganisms, pollution, and other environmental toxins. In the aftermath of the devastation from the atomic bomb explosion in Hiroshima, Japan, in 1945, the first green plant shoots to appear were those of *Ginkgo biloba*. Today these hardy trees line many of the busy streets of some of the world's largest and most polluted cities, including Tokyo and New York City. The ginkgo tree embodies Darwin's evolutionary theory of the survival of the fittest, enduring for all of these years without mutation; this is another testament to its hardiness.

In China, the ginkgo tree was called *yinhsing*, meaning "silver apricot." The Japanese translation of this was *yin-kwo*, meaning "silver fruit." In English, the ginkgo tree is variously known as the kew tree, fossil tree, or maidenhair tree (after a similarity noted with the fanlike leaves of the true maidenhair tree). Other names for the ginkgo tree include gingo, gingko, ginko, and yin guo.

Revering life and honoring the elderly, the Chinese noted the positive effects of ginkgo long ago. Documentation of these effects dates back to 2700 B.C. (nearly 5,000 years ago!), when an ancient Chinese herbal medical text noted that ginkgo leaves could reverse memory loss in the elderly and ease breathing problems. In accordance with the Eastern yin and yang philosophy, in traditional Chinese medicine (TCM) practice, ginkgo seeds were deemed "dry" and recommended to treat "wet" conditions such as asthma, chronic diarrhea, and peripheral (hand or foot) swelling due to cold damp exposure. Roasted seeds were used as a digestive aid and were believed to prevent drunkenness.

Indeed, ginkgo seeds have been used for centuries in TCM. They have been prescribed as treatments for memory decline with aging, asthma, cough, cystitis (bladder inflammation), mucous discharge, vaginal discharge, and alcohol abuse. To this day, ginkgo seeds are frequently included on celebration menus in China and Japan, on occasions when people are likely to eat and drink to excess, to counteract the effects of overindulging. We don't know how this works, but perhaps it is related to ginkgo's enhancement of blood flow, which could thereby improve digestive function. While not a part of TCM, ginkgo leaves are prescribed in Chinese popular medicine, with applications in treating asthma, pulmonary tuberculosis, vaginal discharge, and problems with sperm production, as well as anginal chest pain, hypercholesterolemia, intestinal inflammation, and filarial or nemotode worm infections.

By the 15th century, ginkgo was used widely in TCM practices throughout China to promote the health and well-being of the brain and lungs and to treat respiratory symptoms, such as coughs and wheezing, as well as parasitic infections. But it was not until the 18th century that the ginkgo tree was made known to the West, by Englebert Kaempfer, a German physician and botanist, who encountered the tree on a 1712 trip to Japan, where he recorded its medicinal uses in his writings. The tree was first brought to Europe in 1730, where it was planted in Holland. By the 19th century the tree was growing widely in Europe's large cities and was well-known enough to be mentioned in the writings of popular authors such as Oliver Wendell Holmes and Sir Arthur Conan Doyle. The ginkgo tree was brought to America soon after the Revolutionary War. It was first planted in Philadelphia but now grows throughout the United States.

Today, *Gingko biloba* is widely used in Germany and France, where it is one of the most common medications prescribed by doctors. It is also one of the most widely used over-the- counter medications, available without prescription in lower dosage formulations.

Today the ginkgo tree grows around the world, thriving in sunny climates and average soil. The bulk herb is produced predominantly in China, Japan, North and South Korea, southern France, and North America. It is the leaf component that is harvested, dried, and used to produce the crude drug that is processed to yield the marketed standardized extract. In contrast to the seed preparations used in TCM, only leaf extracts are used for medicinal purposes in Europe.

How Ginkgo Is Used as a Remedy Today

In Germany, where herbal remedies are widely accepted, ginkgo was approved in 1991 for the treatment of a number of specific conditions:

- Ginkgo is used widely to treat memory and other cognitive impairments that come with dementia, whether related to impaired blood supply, to a primary degenerative condition such as Alzheimer's disease, or to both. Symptoms used to guide treatment in these areas include memory deficits, poor concentration, depression, dizziness, ringing in the ears, and headache.
- Ginkgo is also used as part of a treatment regimen for a condition called *intermittent claudication*, whereby blockage of peripheral arteries leads to leg pain when one is walking.
- Other conditions for which ginkgo is approved are vertigo and ringing in the ears, also called *tinnitus*, whether related to vascular or other causes.

What could ginkgo's remedial powers mean for those of us struggling to stay sharp in our day-to-day functioning? Ginkgo can be used by adults, young and old ones alike, with potential benefits ranging from improved alertness, attention, and memory in healthy individuals; to cognitive enhancement in the elderly; to mild, but potentially important, benefits in those with more significant dementing illness.

Tim, age 21, is in his junior year of college. He plans to pursue a career in marketing but first needs to cross the hurdle of getting into business school. His grades had been pretty good, but as he was studying for the GMAT exam he found he was having more trouble than usual keeping on top of things. Concerned that his grades would slip and wanting to stay very focused for the exam, he started taking 120 mg of *Ginkgo biloba* twice per day before tests and paper deadlines. Over the course of the semester he was very pleased with his performance, noting "a dramatic improvement in my grades, including several top papers," and scoring in the 98th percentile on the verbal component of the GMAT. Last spring he was accepted to his top graduate school choice, and he continues to use ginkgo without any adverse effects.

Bob is a 68-year-old widower who was has had memory problems for more than 10 years. His problems started several years ago after an accident at work that resulted in his exposure to dangerous levels of carbon monoxide. He was never the same after the accident. He became profoundly depressed and developed significant memory problems and severe headaches. His cognitive function never fully returned, and he ultimately became disabled and had his driver's license revoked. We found his depression very difficult to treat; he responded poorly to a variety of treatments, including electroconvulsive therapy and multiple trials of antidepressants. Eventually he tried a regimen of the antidepressant medication Celexa (citalopram), as well as *Ginkgo biloba*, at a dosage of 120 mg twice per day. He thought he noted some improvement after several weeks, but after two months on the regimen he definitely felt "the best I have been in a long, long time." He was clearly more alert, and his concentration and memory were significantly better. Today he is once again enjoying life and continues to live independently, even more so after regaining his driver's license last spring.

Betty is an 82-year-old retired goverment employee. She has been happily married for 60 years and had been very successful in her job right up to retirement. Over an eight-month period her family noted progressive changes in her behavior and trouble with her memory. According to her husband, on a number of occasions she had driven to a distant hotel, but was unable to recall how she got there or why she was there. Concerned for her safety, the family took away her driver's license. At times she would become paranoid when seeing her reflection in a mirror, mistaking it for an intruder in the house. Despite all this, she remained very pleasant and sociable. When she came to see us, she was clearly confused and disoriented. Her immediate recall was extremely poor, and she did not know the date or where she was. After making a thorough evaluation, we diagnosed her with dementia, and started her on a prescription medication, Aricept (donazepil). Unfortunately, after several months of treatment, her condition was essentially unchanged; indeed, she actually manifested further deterioration in her judgment. We then tried Betty on a trial of *Ginkgo biloba*, initially at 180 mg per day and later at 240 mg daily. At follow-up six months later, she was doing a bit better, which was particularly remarkable since in the interim her husband had died and she had moved into an assisted living complex. Nonetheless, she noted more energy, was playing golf regularly, and in general was adjusting fairly well to the loss of her lifelong companion and to her new living environment. Her cognitive function was remarkably stable, without further deterioration.

To understand how ginkgo helped such diverse people as Tim, Bob, and Betty—and how it might help you too, with mental decline and other problems—you need to know a little about the processes that affect our bodies and our minds as we age. Some of these processes are a normal part of growing older, while others are not necessarily "normal" even though they may be quite common.

The Effects of Aging on the Body

It may be hard to believe, but by our early twenties—a time when most people feel full of life, embarking on the challenges and excitement of adulthood—the aging process has already started. Blood flow to the brain begins to decrease, albeit very slowly; it may take more effort to learn new things; and our reaction time begins to diminish. By age 25, many women are beginning to lose calcium from their bones. Further changes occur naturally and gradually over the next 30 to 40 years and affect every organ system in the body. These processes can be accelerated by environmental and lifestyle factors such as smoking, poor diet, lack of exercise, excessive weight gain, alcohol or drug abuse, and excessive sun exposure. Betty was beginning to feel the effects of aging on the brain, but, surprisingly, so was Tim. Bob's condition had a number of causes, with the toxic effects of carbon monoxide poisoning and oxygen deprivation being allied to the physiological changes that occur in the sixth decade of life.

Physiological Changes Associated with Aging

Blood Vessels

(1) Loss of elasticity and increased resistance to normal blood flow in vessels. (2) Deposition of plaques and other debris, leading to formation of clots. These changes lead to a reduction in blood flow, insufficient blood supply to vital bodily organs, and inadequate oxygenation and nourishment of cells and tissues. These alterations ultimately have an impact on all organs in the body, including the brain, heart, lungs, kidneys, liver, gastrointestinal tract, endocrine glands, reproductive system, sensory organs, muscles, bones, skin, and hematopoietic system (which makes new blood cells).

Nervous System

(1) Reduction in number of nerve cells in the brain and in overall mass of the brain. (2) Reduction in number of peripheral nerve fibers (those supplying sites outside the brain and regulating both voluntary activities, such as walking and feeding, and involuntary ones, such as breathing and hearing). (3) Slowing in velocity of nerve cell conduction, so that it takes longer for the signal to get there. (4) Reduced blood supply to the nerves, leading to nerve cell injury and death. This occurs very

commonly in the brain, which in its innermost regions is supplied by the blood vessels that are smallest and farthest away from the larger, primary blood vessels, and leads to a condition called *cerebral insufficiency*. (5) Decline in function of sensory organs, with visual deterioration, hearing loss, and reduction in sharpness of the senses of smell and taste.

Cardiovascular

(1) With changes in properties of blood vessels, vessels become more rigid and inflexible, and are apt to sustain higher internal pressures (e.g., high blood pressure, or hypertension). (2) Inadequate blood supply to the heart muscle results in heart muscle injury and ultimately deterioration in heart function. (3) Reduced blood flow to peripheral sites, such are hands and feet, can affect the nerves supplying these areas, leading to sensory changes such as numbness and tingling and, in more severe cases, can lead to ischemic changes (tissue damage) necessitating amputation of the affected areas.

Metabolic

(1) Reduction in the body's metabolic rate. (2) Loss of muscle mass and increase in body fat content, with resultant alterations in how substances we ingest are metabolized.

Endocrinologic

(1) Changes in endocrine organ (e.g., thyroid gland, pancreas) function can lead to conditions such as hypo- or hyperthyroidism, or diabetes. (2) In women, the loss of estrogen production that occurs with menopause is accompanied by physiological changes affecting multiple organ systems.

Musculoskeletal

(1) Chronic inflammatory states such as arthritis. (2) Osteoporotic changes resulting from loss of bone density, which lead to more delicate bones and increased susceptibility to broken bones such as of the hip and spine, resulting in difficulty walking and alterations in body posture. (3) Longer healing time for injuries.

Skin

(1) Tendency to become thin, with less resilience and elasticity. (2) Longer healing time for injuries. (3) The cumulative effects of years of sun exposure (related to free radicals generated by the effects of sun's radiation) can lead to precancerous or cancerous changes.

The Effects of Aging on Cognition

While it can be frustrating and annoying, some degree of memory loss is a normal accompaniment of aging. It can begin subtly as early as our third and fourth decades, and gradually become more apparent as time wears on to our sixth decade and beyond. These changes are commonly referred to as *age-related memory decline* or *loss*.

Some people, however, experience more severe losses of memory, powers of reasoning, and judgment. These changes can have a significant impact on their day-to-day functioning and quality of life and all too often leave them dependent on their loved ones. Such changes are seen in dementia and are sadly often the harbinger of further deterioration and loss of independence. While such forms of mental decline are not normal, they are becoming increasingly common as our senior population grows in numbers.

Clearly, some of the most profound and debilitating effects observed with aging can be those associated with mental functioning or cognition: the ability to consider, evaluate, and make appropriate responses to internal and external stimuli. Aging can rob us of the ability to pay attention, to orient ourselves in our world, to learn new things and remember old ones, to comprehend and make judgments, to use language, to organize our motor skills, to interpret sensations, and to make skilled movements with accuracy, such as correctly drawing the face of a clock or dressing ourselves. These changes can be attributed to a number of physiological alterations that occur when we get older.

Disruption of the Blood–Brain Barrier

The blood–brain barrier, a natural membranous shield encasing the central nervous system (CNS; including the brain and spinal cord), is comprised of a network of tissue and delicate capillaries across which oxygen, glucose, and other nutrients are delivered to the CNS and waste products removed. These capillary vessels thicken with age, thereby interfering with the delivery and removal processes and becoming leaky, allowing the entry of unwanted substances that can disrupt the delicate biochemical balance in the CNS. Such biochemical imbalances may contribute to the increased susceptibility to medication side effects that we see in the elderly.

Cerebral Insufficiency

Diminished blood flow to nerve cells in the brain compromises the brain's supply of important nutrients, particularly oxygen and glucose, and results in a condition called *cerebral insufficiency*. A number of problems commonly reported in the elderly have been associated with cerebral insufficiency, including memory difficulty, poor concentration and distractibility, confusion, lethargy, fatigue, weakness, anxiety, depression, ringing in the ears, and headache. In some cases these symptoms represent early stages of the dementing process or some other degenerative condition. These symptoms, however, may also appear subtly in middle age and become more evident over the years. Adults in their forties and fifties, often beset with the challenge of caring for not-yet-grown children and aging parents of their own, can find themselves under additional stress when they start forgetting appointments and losing the ability to juggle several mental tasks at once. These changes are, however, subtle. Most of us simply adapt without really knowing it. It's when others—for example, doctors, family members—start noticing that we are functioning at less than our normal capacity that a more significant problem such as the onset of dementia may be occurring.

Memory Loss

By the time we are in our sixth or seventh decade, what started as annoying but normal forgetfulness may have progressed to more pervasive memory difficulty, with trouble learning new information and recalling recent events, while more remote memories frequently remain intact. These changes may be associated with a medical problem, such as hypothyroidism, or with other conditions such as depression or anxiety, but they can also be part of progressive intellectual impairment due to a decline in certain neurochemicals in the brain as well as the destruction of nerve cells by free radicals (see box on page 179) in the memory centers of the brain.

Dementia

Dementia is a condition characterized by progressive, persistent decline in cognitive functioning. Over time these cognitive changes can lead to a more global impairment, with deterioration in intellectual, emotional, and behavioral capacities, resulting in a decline in overall functioning. The overwhelming majority of causes of dementia are irreversible.

The most common causes of dementia are Alzheimer's disease (AD) and cerebrovascular disease. The cause of AD is unknown, but it does seem to have a genetic component because it often runs in families. It usually strikes in the sixth and seventh decades, slowly and steadily progressing to the point where its victims are unable to live independently and care for themselves. But AD can also affect younger people, with onset in the fifties; however, this is a much rarer variant of the illness. At this point the only way we can make a definitive diagnosis of AD is through examination of brain tissue on autopsy, where the neurofibrillary plaques and tangles characteristic of the disease can be identified under a microscope. While we can in theory perform this test on a living individual in whom we suspect AD, the risks associated with taking a sample of brain tissue from a live person are not outweighed by the benefits of making a definitive diagnosis of what remains an incurable illness. Hopefully, this will change with time, as we develop a better understanding of the cause(s) of AD and develop treatments and maybe even preventive strategies for the disease.

The other common type of dementia is called multi-infarct dementia (MID) or vascular dementia, because it is caused by changes that occur over many years in the blood vessels supplying the brain. These changes are often related to the long-term effects of a number of chronic medical conditions that affect blood vessels, such as high blood pressure, heart disease, diabetes, and alcoholism. While the cognitive decline may be less insidious with MID, sufferers often have to contend with the aftereffects of these other serious medical conditions, problems that often include strokes, heart attacks and weakened heart function, kidney problems, blindness, difficulty walking, and poor balance.

While this picture may develop from a variety of causes, the common denominator in all these processes is their impact on the blood supply to the brain and directly on neural tissue. As such, the final common pathway is the destruction of brain tissue through the deprivation of oxygen and other nutrients, depletion of proteins, and other damage (e.g., free radical injury; see box on page 179). A variety of other medical conditions, such as vitamin B_{12} deficiency or depression, may cause similar symptoms, but in these cases the cognitive impairment is usually reversible following the appropriate diagnosis and treatment. Characteristic symptoms of dementia are listed in Table 10.

Table 10. Characteristic Symptoms of Dementia

- Development of multiple cognitive deficits manifested by memory impairment and other cognitive disturbances:
  - Disturbance in language abilities (i.e., aphasia)
  - Problems performing activities in spite of normal motor function (i.e., apraxia)
  - Difficulty recognizing or identifying objects in spite of normal sensory function (i.e., agnosia)
  - Problems with executive functions of planning, organizing, sequencing, abstracting
- Significant interference by these deficits with normal day to day functioning, representing a significant decline from previous functioning
- Gradual onset of symptoms and progressive decline in functioning
- Changes not caused by another CNS or medical or mental condition causing similar deficits
- Changes not occurring exclusively during the course of a delirium

Note. Adapted with permission from the *Diagnostic and Statistical Manual for Mental Disorders*, fourth edition. Copyright 1994 by the American Psychiatric Association.

What Ginkgo Does to Fight the Effects of Aging and Injury

So, how does ginkgo combat these multifarious effects of aging (and also injury)? One way it does so is by neutralizing free radicals, those electron-challenged raiders to which we are all exposed during life via various environmental toxins and radiation—even life-giving sunlight. Free radicals are particularly fond of attacking one of the components of nerve cells, such as brain cells, and play a major role in the physiological changes that come with aging—whether at the beginning of the aging process, as in Tim's case, or at the later stages of the process, as in Betty's case. Free radicals can also cause severe damage, such as in response to the toxic carbon monoxide that injured Bob.

But there's more: While certain ingredients in ginkgo are scavenging the free radicals that attack an important element in brain cells, other ingredients are helping the body produce that very element in the precise region of the brain involved in memory. That is, ginkgo not only attacks the free radicals that destroy brain cells but helps to nourish and restore those cells in the memory centers of the brain.

And, believe it or not, ginkgo also strengthens capillary walls and offsets clotting, thereby increasing the flow of blood and delivery of oxygen the brain needs. That means it can not only fight a significant effect of aging but also help a young adult get closer to peak brain function.

We're excited about ginkgo's potential to improve the quality of life for all of us because through the same mechanisms of action it can either heal damage done to the body by injury or disease or combat the more insidious, gradual tissue and vessel changes that come with age. Of course, in many ways it's all the same type of damage, whether caused by injury, illness, or time.

Let's see what the scientific research has shown us about what ginkgo may be able to do for cognitive function, how the herb compares to alternative treatments, and what else this flexible herb seems to offer to our health. More detail on ginkgo's mechanisms of action can be found under "How Ginkgo Works" on page 177.

Treating Cognitive Problems with Ginkgo

Ginkgo has been used and studied most widely as a treatment for the memory decline and cognitive deficits seen with aging. In Europe, these changes are classified under the rubric of "cerebral insufficiency"; in the United States, these symptoms are referred to as "age-associated memory impairment." In the last 20 years numerous controlled clinical trials of ginkgo have been performed, predominantly in Germany and France, and the results are promising. Many of these reports have suggested that ginkgo helps to improve or slow down the impairment observed in people with dementia and to improve aging-related memory decline. As we'll discuss in more detail on page 177, ginkgo most likely helps the brain and cognitive functioning in a number of ways, through enhanced blood flow, improved oxygen and glucose delivery, and scavenging of toxic free radicals, thereby protecting nerve cells and blood vessels.

Memory Impairment and Dementia

Over the last 20 years, more than 50 clinical trials have demonstrated efficacy for ginkgo in cerebral insufficiency and dementia. Naturally, however, not all studies met the same standards for rigorous design and control, and it is important to keep this in mind when interpreting the results.

Trials of ginkgo in cerebral insufficiency have been critically reviewed in two comprehensive reports. In a critical review of 40 clinical trials, Kleijnen and Knipschild (1992) identified eight trials that met their qualifications for good study methodology. All but one of these trials showed positive effects for ginkgo, in doses of 120 to 160 mg per day over 12 weeks, but benefits were not really discernable until at least week 6. Overall, 70 percent of those receiving ginkgo improved compared to 14 percent of those on placebo. No serious side effects were reported, and those noted did not differ between individuals taking ginkgo and those taking placebo. A second review of 11 placebo-controlled studies conducted by Hopfenmuller (1994) published in the respected German medical journal *Arzneimittelforschung* also found ginkgo to be effective in combating cerebral insufficiency.

In another comprehensive review, Oken and his colleagues (1998) examined over 50 articles reporting on ginkgo's effect on cognitive function in patients with mild to moderate dementia related to AD. In the four studies that met their criteria for minimally acceptable scientific standards, a total of 424 subjects had been treated, half of whom received 120 to 240 mg per day of standardized ginkgo extract and the other half a placebo equivalent. After three to six months of treatment, small but significant improvements were observed in cognitive function, and treatment was well tolerated.

Since the publication of these reviews, findings from several other large placebo-controlled trials of standardized ginkgo extract in dementia have been reported. Findings from a large well-controlled study of patients with mild to severe dementia from AD or MID performed in the United States were published in the *Journal of the American Medical Association*. In their report, Le Bars and his colleagues (1998) described their findings from a 52-week randomized, double-blind, placebo-controlled multicenter trial—the "gold standard" type of medication study. Three hundred nine outpatients with mild to severe AD or MID were treated with either 120 mg per day of standardized ginkgo extract or placebo for one year. They were evaluated every three months with assessments of cognitive function using three standardized scales. Two hundred twelve subjects were included in the data analysis at one year. Modest but significant improvements in cognitive functioning and social performance were observed in those receiving ginkgo as measured by changes in two of the scales. No significant changes, however, were observed in the doctor's clinical assessment—not a terribly surprising finding since the changes may have been subtle and not detectable by a doctor examining the patient at isolated time points. Ginkgo was well tolerated, and no differences were observed in side effects reported in the two groups.

In another study performed in Germany, Kanowski et al. (1997) also compared the effects of ginkgo against placebo in 216 patients with mild to moderate AD or MID. Over the course of a year, patients were treated with either 240 mg of ginkgo extract or placebo daily. Patient improvement was evaluated using standardized ratings for attention and memory, behavioral function in activities of daily living (ADLs), and a doctor's assessment of overall improvement. After one year of treatment, patients treated with ginkgo showed significant improvement over those receiving placebo in each of these areas. Furthermore, ginkgo was well tolerated.

Information pooled in careful literature reviews, as well as information from high-quality individual studies, can give us a good overall picture of the subject being studied. Together, these findings on ginkgo demonstrate that the herb appears safe and effective in treating mild to moderate symptoms of dementia. When compared to placebo, significant improvements are observed with ginkgo. *While these differences often corresponded to relatively small clinical changes, in a condition that leads to progressive and inevitable deterioration even a relatively brief delay in this degenerative process can be very important.* Many questions remain: perhaps ginkgo may be of greater benefit when used in concert with prescription medications; or perhaps it can be more effective, maybe even preventive, when taken earlier in life.

Normal Memory

Can ginkgo really help people like Tim, the student we described earlier, improve their overall mental performance by sharpening their memory? Though this topic has been less widely studied, ginkgo has been associated with memory improvement in healthy people. In a study by Rai et al. (1991) conducted in England, 31 adults over age 50 with mild memory loss were treated with 120 mg per day of standardized ginkgo extract or placebo. At evaluation after 12 and 24 months of treatment, adults receiving ginkgo had better cognitive function and quicker response time. In another small study by Hindmarch (1986) of short-term memory, eight healthy women between the ages of 25 and 40 were treated with ginkgo, receiving 120 to 600 mg of ginkgo or placebo equivalent. One hour later, they were administered a battery of memory tests. Short-term memory was improved significantly in subjects receiving the 600-mg dose, while changes in the other groups were no different from placebo. Another study assessed the acute effects of ginkgo or placebo one hour after dosing administration (Warot et al., 1991) but found essentially no differences between treatments. While it is hard to know exactly what to make of these results given the very small number of participants, they are intriguing findings and warrant further investigation.

A third study (Rigney et al., 1999) looked at the acute effects of ginkgo on memory and psychomotor performance in 31 healthy volunteers, aged 30 to 59 years. This randomized double-blind crossover study compared the effects of four different doses of ginkgo (50 mg three times per day, 100 mg three times per day, 120 mg per day, and 240 mg per day) against placebo; participants received each treatment for two days. A battery of tests was administered prior to treatment and at frequent intervals until 11 hours post dose. Analysis of the test results revealed that ginkgo was effective for memory, particularly working memory, with the most substantial effects observed at the 120 mg dose. Interestingly, the authors noted further that the cognitive enhancing effects were most likely to be apparent in the 50 to 59 age group.

Other Treatments for Cognitive Impairments

How do other treatments compare to ginkgo in treating cognitive decline? Dementia has multiple causes leading to the same end point, and our knowledge base in this area is limited. The research is very expensive to conduct, and the results of medical treatments to date have not been terribly impressive. All this adds up to slow progress toward reversing or preventing the impairments in mental functioning caused by aging and disease.

Pharmaceutical Treatments

To date only two medications have been approved in the United States for treating the cognitive decline seen in AD (see Table 11). These drugs, Tacrine (tetrahydroaminoacridine) and Aricept (donepezil), inhibit the enzyme acetylcholinesterase, which prevents the breakdown of choline, an important neurotransmitter involved in memory functions, thereby making choline more available at nerve endings, where it facilitates processes that contribute to memory functioning. The other three agents listed in the table have not been approved by the FDA for this use. Other treatments under investigation have included velnacrine maleate, acetyl L-carnitine, lecithin, 4-aminopyridine, arecholine, phoshpati-

Table 11. Treatments for Dementia

Drug (generic name)	Mechanism	Results
Tacrine (tetrahydroaminoacridine)	Cholinesterase inhibitor	Equivocal improvement in performance-based tests, global assessments by clinicians and caregivers, and quality of life; potential for liver toxicity. Not approved for use in some countries because the risks of toxicity outweigh the benefits to cognition.
Aricept (donepezil)	Cholinesterase inhibitor	Significant improvement observed in certain cognitive parameters, but not in functional abilities, quality of life, caregiver burden, and overall disease severity. Some evidence suggests it may reduce the rate of cognitive decline, but further study is needed.
Eldepryl (selegiline hydrochloride)	MAO B inhibitor	In small studies, some improvement in cognitive test scores, information handling, and independence in ADLs, but not clinically significant.
Hydergine (dihydroergotoxine)	Beta-adrenergic, dopaminergic, and serotonergic activity	A combination of ergoloid mesylates around since the 1940s, it affects several neurotransmitter systems in the central nervous system. Findings from clinical trials have been inconclusive.
Vitamin E	Antioxidant	In a study comparing this with selegiline, vitamin E delayed time to occurrence of death, institutionalization, loss of ability to perform ADLs, or severe dementia. However, it was associated with increased rate of dizziness and falls when compared to placebo. No benefits when combined with selegiline. Only after statistical adjustments did either treatment show a significant advantage.

Note. ADLs, activities of daily living.

dylserine, memantine, naloxone hydrochloride, nimodipine, aniracetam, and propentofylline.

Clinical trials have shown improvement in cognition in patients with mild to moderate Alzheimer's-type dementia treated with Tacrine compared to placebo, but this improvement is not dramatic. Also, some people have developed liver problems when taking the drug (although these problems usually resolve once the medication is stopped). Aricept has also shown some benefit in people with mild to moderate dementia attributable to AD. It is generally well tolerated, with only occasional reports of side effects, usually noted at higher doses, including nausea, diarrhea, and vomiting. Generally only a minority of individuals will report some symptomatic relief with these treatments, and in some cases the side effects have outweighed the benefits of the treatment.

Traditional Herbal Remedies

As we continue to learn more about the brain and the mechanisms related to normal memory decline and to the pathological development of dementia, we hope we will be better armed to develop new treatments that are safe and effective. Such treatments may very well include herbal remedies besides ginkgo. Medical traditions in the Far East and India have recognized the cognitive- and memory-enhancing ability of plants for centuries, though ginkgo has consistently emerged as the frontrunner.

We are really just beginning to understand how some of these plant extracts affect memory and cognitive function. Our knowledge of these mechanisms should improve with time, as we develop a greater understanding of the biological underpinnings of dementia. Medicinal plants that enhance transmission of specific neurotransmitters may potentially act to reduce free radical activity and inflammation, prevent the formation of and toxicity related to destructive proteins such as B-amyloid, and increase levels of substances that promote nerve health, including estrogen. As such, medicinal plants may well help to open the way for understanding of new mechanisms and treatments. Table 12 lists plants other than ginkgo that have been used for their cognitive-enhancing effects in different cultures.

The memory-enhancing effects of many plants are supported by evidence from experience dating back through hundreds of years of recorded history. For example, lemon balm has been reported as "sovereign for the brain, strengthening the memory and powerfully chasing away the melancholy" (John Evelyn, 1699). Sage was reported to be "singularly good for the head and brain and quickeneth the nerves and memory" (John Gerard,

Table 12. Herbs with Cognitive-Enhancing Effects

Plant	Activity	Uses
Paeony (*Paeonia suffruticosa*)	Cholinergic	Component of traditional Chinese herbal prescriptions for dementia such as jin gui shen qi wen and lui wei di huang wan. Improves performance in rats treated with scopolamine; anti-anmestic properties and cortical cholinergic activity.
Angelica (*Angelica sinensis*)	Cholinesterase inhibitor	Combined with paeony in Shimotsuto and reverses scopolamine-induced performance deficits. Used in China and Japan. May be related to the European *Angelica archangelica* which has nicotinic activity.
Evodia rutarcarpa	Cholinesterase inhibitor	Used in TCM.
Huperzine (*Huperzia serrata*)	Cholinesterase and acetylcholinesterase inhibitor	Derived from a moss, it has traditionally been used to treat inflammation and fever, but is now also used in China to treat dementia.
Mentat	Cholinergic	An Ayurvedic formulation containing 26 plant species
Trasina	Cholinergic	An Ayurvedic formulation of five plant species.
Indian ginseng (*Withania sonmifera*)	Cholinergic, muscarinic	In an animal model, reduced cerebral deficits with inhibition of acetylcholinesterase and enhanced binding to M1-muscarinic receptors.
Korean ginseng (*Panax ginseng*)	Cholinergic	Among its many reported benefits, it is considered to improve memory.
Lemon balm (*Mellisa officinalis*)	Acetylcholinesterase inhibitor; nicotinic receptor inhibition	*In vitro* effects observed; monoterpenes believed to be active chemical and concentrates in the hippocampus (brain area associated with learning and affected in early Alzheimer's disease).
Rosemary (*Rosemary officinalis*)	?	Used in the United Kingdom by medical herbalists and aromatherapists for memory problems.
Sage (*Salvia officinalis*)	Acetylcholinesterase inhibitor; nicotinic receptor inhibition	Similar properties observed in other *Salvia* species, which may have a lower risk for toxicity. Used in TCM, Ayurvedic medicine, and European herbal medicine since the 1500s.

(continued)

Table 12 (continued)

Plant	Activity	Uses
Calabar bean (*Physostigma venenosa*)	Cholinesterase inhibitor	Active chemical is physostigmine which is not traditionally known for use in memory enhancement. From West Africa, it was used as a purgative in witchcraft trials.
Snowgrop (*Galanthus nivalis*), Daffodil (*Narcissus*)	Cholinesterase inhibitor	In one study, significantly improved symptoms in patients with Alzheimer's disease, but can also be associated with substantial nausea and vomiting.
Guarana (*Paullinia cupana, P. sorbilis*)	Stimulant	Native to the Amazon Basin in Brazil, this plant has been used locally for centuries as a tonic and a stimulant. Contains methylxanthine alkaloids, but its effects are believed to be through its high caffeine content—up to almost four times that found in coffee beans or dried tea leaves. There is little clinical evidence to support its safety and efficacy in enhancing mental performance. There are potentially serious safety concerns given possible carcinogenic effects related to a high tannin content, as well as a highly variable caffeine content.

Note. Some data are from Perry et al. (1999).

1597). Even Shakespeare alluded to the memory-enhancing effects of herbs, when in *Hamlet* the character Ophelia declares, "There's rosemary; that's for remembrance. Pray, love, remember."

Scientific data, however, are derived from findings from animal models and a very limited database from controlled clinical studies. A handful of controlled trials have demonstrated effects for huperzia, narcissus, *panax ginseng*, and *physostigma venenosa*, in addition to ginkgo. Particular interest has recently developed regarding huperzine, with some researchers believing that it may be more effective than either Tacrine or Aricept. Huperzine appears to have greater binding activity to important CNS sites than either drug, with a longer half-life and fewer side effects, and may also reduce glutamate-induced nerve cell death. Positive results from controlled studies are encouraging, but further investigation of safety and efficacy is needed.

A Combined Approach

Not surprisingly, lifestyle factors that increase blood flow and promote blood vessel strength can help to keep mental powers sharp. For example, exercise, dietary habits that help to offset processes that lead to clogged blood vessels, and avoidance of dietary and environmental sources of free radicals can all contribute to enduring memory and alertness. In general, these important factors relate to living a balanced lifestyle: all things in moderation. So, as we suggest for fighting depression (Chapter 1), stress and anxiety (Chapter 2), and insomnia (Chapter 4), a multipronged approach to fighting cognitive decline may be best of all.

Ginkgo and Other Parts of the Body

Does its ability to slow the effects of aging on the brain qualify ginkgo for the title "fountain of youth"? Perhaps not. But when its other felicitous effects are taken into account, ginkgo seems like a natural wonder indeed! After all, there are no synthetic or other known natural products with the range of clinical applications that we see in ginkgo.

Circulation

When the body's tissues, particularly in the heart and brain, have been temporarily deprived of oxygen, for example, as in vessel blockage leading to transient ischemic attacks (TIAs) and strokes, or in narrowing caused by vasospasm, or in toxicity resulting from inadequate oxygen supply, toxic free radicals are generated and tissue damage follows. As we explain on pages 178–181, ginkgo may help in these circumstances both because it is a free radical "scavenger" and because it helps vessels relax, thereby promoting improved blood flow and enhanced delivery of oxygen and glucose.

The Heart and the Major Blood Vessels. In both animal models and *in vitro* models using human endothelial cells (i.e., cells lining vessel walls), ginkgo has been shown to protect the heart muscle and blood vessels from injury. Ginkgo has also prevented tissue injury following reconstructive surgery in rats. The effects observed here are likely due to the combined effects of the various components of the ginkgo, not just to a single constituent.

Ginkgo may protect the heart and blood vessels in humans too. In a report published in 1997, a group of investigators in France (Pietri et al., 1997) described a study of patients undergoing aortic heart valve replacement surgery. This procedure requires that the blood be rerouted away from the heart and lungs during the surgery before being returned to these organs when normal blood flow is restored. For five days before the procedure, eight patients received 320 mg per day of standardized ginkgo extract and seven received a placebo equivalent. Blood samples were collected at specific intervals during and up to eight days following the surgery. A number of differences were noted in the blood samples related to the activity of free radicals. Although the difference was not statistically significant, patients receiving ginkgo generally did better than those receiving placebo.

Peripheral Circulation. Ginkgo has also demonstrated beneficial effects on circulation in both the large (i.e., arteries and veins) and small (i.e., capillary) blood vessels. In an open study of people with long histories of circulatory problems, Witte et al. (1992) treated 20 outpatients with 240 mg per day of ginkgo for 12 weeks. Following treatment, patients' fibrinogen levels were significantly reduced and blood flow properties improved. Fibrinogen is a substance that is a part of our body's normal blood-clotting mechanism but that also accumulates in response to injury, for example, from certain trauma and physiological insults. The authors thereby proposed that with these changes ginkgo could have a positive effect on this cardiovascular risk factor (i.e., circulatory problems)over time. In a placebo-controlled crossover study in 10 healthy volunteers, when compared to placebo, treatment with ginkgo was associated with improvement in blood fluidity and capillary microcirculation (Jung et al., 1990).

Impairment in the peripheral arterial blood supply can lead to sensations of cold and numbness, leg cramping, and a condition called *intermittent claudication* characterized by significant leg pain with walking. As the condition worsens, the person's activity can be limited substantially as the pain increases over shorter distances. In 1992 Schneider (1992) performed a meta-analysis that examined the utility of ginkgo in treating these conditions. Results from five placebo-controlled clinical trials were examined. He found that with ginkgo patients were able to walk longer distances more comfortably, with significant pain relief. In addition, these benefits often persisted for several months following the discontinuation of treatment.

Ginkgo and the Senses

As we age, we observe changes in our senses, with a gradual decline in function: annoying ringing in the ears, or tinnitus, may develop; you must ask people to repeat themselves because you cannot hear them; vision may need correction with eyeglasses; and unsteadiness may develop, with a disturbance in balance and equilibrium. Recent studies indicate that ginkgo, with its antioxidant and vasoprotective activities, may actually be helpful in improving these common effects of aging.

Tinnitus. Several studies have shown that ginkgo can be effective in reducing tinnitus, persistent ringing in the ears that in many cases is caused by poor circulation in the brain. In one double-blind, placebo-controlled trial, patients with tinnitus for less than one year were treated with either 320 mg per day of ginkgo or a placebo. After one month, greater improvement was observed among subjects taking ginkgo. While the tinnitus persisted, it was at least diminished if not more substantially improved (Meyer, 1986). We should point out that the symptoms were of relatively short duration, at less than one year, and it is possible that similar effects may not have been observed in subjects with more long-standing symptoms.

Findings from another study suggest that ginkgo may also help early hearing loss due to damage to the cochlear nerve, that is, damage to the nerve supplying impulses to the inner ear where sounds waves are transmuted into nerve impulses. In a placebo-controlled trial by Dubreuil (1986) subjects were treated with either ginkgo or a medication that blocks a specific neurotransmitter, an alpha-blocker (nicergoline). Significant improvement was demonstrated in both groups but was greater with ginkgo.

Balance and Equilibrium. Balance and orientation are complex processes receiving neural inputs from our eyes, from sensory nerves that help to orient us in space, and from our inner ears where equilibrium is interpreted, with the brain's cerebellum acting as the central processor. Impaired blood flow to the nerves supplying any of these regions can cause problems with balance. Over the last two decades several studies have suggested that ginkgo may help to offset these symptoms. In a double-blind multicenter study by Haguenauer et al. (1986), 70 patients with new onset imbalance of unknown cause were treated for three months, after which time 47 percent of those taking ginkgo were without symptoms compared to 18 percent of placebo controls. It should be noted that the balance disturbances studied in this trial were of relatively brief duration and that similar results may not be seen with a more chronic condition. In a more recent controlled study by Cesarani et al. (1998), 44 patients with dizziness and/or vertigo related to vascular inner ear disorders were treated for three months with either ginkgo (80 mg twice per day) or betahistine hydrochloride (16 mg twice a day). A comprehensive battery of tests was performed at baseline and after three months of treatment. A number of improvements were observed with each of the treatments, suggesting that these drugs operate on different receptor sites. In particular, the researchers concluded that ginkgo can considerably improve oculomotor and visuovestibular function. Side effects were rare and both medications were well tolerated.

Retinal Changes. Visual changes with age are related to a multitude of causes: "normal" age-related changes, particularly nearsightedness and farsightedness; long-standing effects of chronic medical conditions affecting blood vessels, such as hypertension, atherosclerosis, and diabetes; and damage from primary ophthalmological conditions, such as glaucoma or macular degeneration. Several of these changes result in injury to the retina, the nerve tissue that lines the inside of the eye. Findings from animal studies have provided preliminary information showing reduced retinal damage following injury in animals receiving ginkgo. These animal studies have provided impetus for further human trials. In one small controlled study of 10 subjects with senile (age-related) macular degeneration (Lebuisson et al., 1986), significant improvement in long-distance visual acuity was observed in those taking ginkgo compared to those taking placebo. These changes were noted in spite of the very small sample. The authors attributed the effects to the antioxidant activity of ginkgo. Another study of 24 elderly adults with chronic cerebral retinal insufficiency tested the effect of ginkgo on the reversibility of visual field deficits. Raabe et al. (1991) found improvement at 160 mg per day, but not at the lower 80 mg per day dose, as assessed individually by patients and their doctors. Furthermore, the retinal areas with more damage were more strongly influenced than healthy areas. The authors concluded that their findings demonstrated reversibility of visual field damage caused by chronic blood flow impairment to the retina.

Visual changes in individuals with diabetes are very frequently related to retinal damage caused by years of poor blood sugar control, leading to a condition called *diabetic retinopathy*. While results from a number of animal studies have suggested that ginkgo may be helpful in this condition, controlled clinical information is limited to findings from one trial. Over a six-month period 29 subjects with early diabetic retinopathy were treated with ginkgo or placebo, and changes in their visual function, including color vision, were assessed (Lanthony and Cosson, 1988). Some improvement, albeit not significant, was observed in those treated with ginkgo, while controls showed a greater rate of decline.

These findings, while limited, offer a ray of hope for those with chronic retinal conditions that carry a significant risk of blindness with progression. Considering that these conditions share blood vessel damage and blood flow impairment, it makes sense that ginkgo might help.

Ginkgo and SSRI-Induced Sexual Dysfunction

There is a small but growing body of information that suggests ginkgo may be helpful in alleviating the sexual dysfunction so commonly reported by men and women taking the SSRI antidepressants. Findings from an open study of 63 patients with sexual dysfunction caused predominantly by SSRIs, Cohen and Bartlik (1998) showed that at doses of 120 to 240 mg per day, ginkgo taken for four to six weeks was associated with significant improvement in sexual functioning. Impressive response rates were noted (75 to 90 percent), with women—for unknown reasons—having a greater response. In our experience, ginkgo can be very effective and is well tolerated but generally needs to be taken in the 180 to 240 mg per day dosage range to be effective. With the herb's safety profile (see page 183), ginkgo may well be a viable solution to this very common and troublesome medication side effect.

Jenny is a 43-year-old travel agent diagnosed with obsessive–compulsive disorder who has responded well to treatment with an SSRI drug. But after a few weeks on Luvox (fluvoxamine) she developed marked difficulty achieving orgasm, and she also noted that her interest in sex had diminished. She was most concerned, however, with her complete inability to achieve orgasm. We advised Jenny to take ginkgo on an as-needed basis, one to two hours ahead of planned sexual activity. This really did not seem to help. So then we suggested four 60-mg tablets per day. After two months on 240 mg of ginkgo per day, Jenny reported that ginkgo had been extraordinarily successful in eliminating the drug-induced side effects. She has continued to take ginkgo for over one year without any loss of effectiveness, provided she takes it every day. Whenever she reduces the frequency, it seems not to be so effective.

Ginkgo and Radiation

We are all exposed to radiation on a daily basis: from the sun, microwaves, televisions, computers, and cellular telephones. Some people are exposed to other types of potentially more harmful radiation as a part of their job—for example, an x-ray technician or someone mining radioactive uranium. At other times, exposure to radiation can be castastrophic, such as the atomic bomb explosion in Hiroshima or the nuclear disaster in Chernobyl, Ukraine, and affect large populations. Radiation decays or breaks down over time, at varying rates and emitting different amounts of energy depending on the source of the radiation. It is this emission of energy, however, that damages cells, by producing free radicals and leading to the production and accumulation of substances called *clastogenic factors* (CFs) that "reprogram" chromosomal DNA on the subatomic level. These changes cause genetic material to mutate and can lead to the production of cancerous cells.

We try to shield ourselves from radiation that might harm us, by using sunscreen, for example, or by having dental x-rays while draped in a lead-lined shield. *Ginkgo biloba* may help to counteract the adverse effects of radiation exposure of which we are unaware. Following the Chernobyl nuclear accident in 1986, workers cleaning up the reactor site were given a thorough medical evaluation. In blood tests, CFs were found in over two-thirds of the workers, indicating that they had been exposed to radiation and were at greater than normal risk of developing cancer over time. Almost a decade later, French investigators (Emerit et al., 1995) conducted a study using ginkgo in these workers, with the hope that ginkgo's antioxidant properties would neutralize the clastogenic factors. Workers were treated with 120 mg per day of standardized ginkgo for two months. Blood samples collected immediately following the treatment period showed clastogenic activity to be at the same level as in nonexposed controls. These benefits persisted on average for at least seven months. But after a year, one-third of the workers again had elevated blood levels of clastogenic activity, demonstrating that the process that generated the CFs continued after discontinuation of ginkgo. Nonetheless, the finding that the herb could confer benefits even when not used continuously is quite intriguing.

Can ginkgo help to counteract the effects of other forms of radiation, such as radiation from the sun? This is a good question. Given the herb's antioxidant activity, it would stand to reason that it may help. Ultraviolet B (UVB) rays seem to cause damage to skin and promote the "aging" process. If ginkgo could neutralize the free radicals produced by UVB exposure, perhaps it could help to deter skin changes related to sun exposure. In a small study looking at the antioxidant effects of several nutritional free radical scavengers in people exposed to controlled amounts of sunshine and ultraviolet light, Pietschmann et al. (1992) found that ginkgo and selenium demonstrated greater antioxidant effects than either beta-carotene or vitamin E. While this is just a preliminary finding, it is certainly intriguing and worthy of further investigation.

Ginkgo and Altitude Sickness

At elevations greater than 9,000 feet, where we are exposed both to colder temperatures and to lower concentrations of oxygen, most people will experience some degree of altitude sickness, which is characterized by dizziness, headache, shortness of breath, nausea, and vomiting. In addition, the colder temperatures can cause constriction of smaller peripheral blood vessels, like those in the microcirculation, and produce symptoms of numbness, tingling, swelling, and pain in our extremities.

In a placebo-controlled study of healthy mountain climbers by Roncin et al. (1996), ginkgo seemed to help protect against these effects. Forty-four subjects who had experienced altitude sickness in the past were randomly assigned to treatment with either 160 mg per day of ginkgo or placebo. Over a period of eight days they climbed to a base camp at 14,700 feet, and thereafter made excursions to higher altitudes. Compared to the placebo group, climbers receiving ginkgo experienced significantly less dizziness and headaches (0 vs. 41 percent) and shortness of breath (14 vs. 82 percent) and were less likely to experience temperature-related symptoms.

Ginkgo and Asthma

Asthma is a respiratory condition characterized by narrowing of the bronchioles, small airway passages in the lungs. As with narrowing of the blood vessels, this narrowing of the bronchioles can have a variety of causes, for example, bronchospasm triggered by exposure to allergens such as pollen or other inhaled pollutants or inflammation and mucous production. In most cases the narrowing produces wheezing and shortness of breath, but in se-

vere cases it can lead to total airway obstruction and death. The role of
ginkgo in mediating these effects has been recognized in China for hundreds of years, where practitioners of TCM have used ginkgo seeds to treat
asthma and bronchitis. In the West, however, it has been only in the last
two decades that interest has developed in this area. Ginkgo's activity is
thought to be related to the herb's antagonism of platelet-activating factor
(PAF) (see page 180), which thereby prevents the cascade of cellular
events leading to inflammation and bronchoconstriction. As we continue
to develop a better understanding of the herb's biochemical activity, we
will likely see more interest in the clinical study of ginkgo's role in mediating the inflammatory and allergic responses seen in asthma.

When You Should *Not* Take Ginkgo

Unless you get a go-ahead from your physician, do not take ginkgo if . . .

- You are taking blood thinners (anticoagulation therapy). If you are
  chronically taking medications that affect platelet activity, such as
  aspirin, talk to your doctor first.
- You have a bleeding or clotting disorder (either inherited disorders
  that cause deficiencies in any of a number of clotting factors, such as
  hemophilia or von Willebrand disease, or acquired disorders, such as
  vitamin K deficiency and other clotting problems that can be associated with liver disease).
- You are pregnant, considering pregnancy, or lactating (breastfeeding). Though Germany's Commission E has said that ginkgo is not
  contraindicated in these populations, you would be wise to consult
  your doctor first.
- You have chronic medical problems requiring regular follow-up and
  medication.

*My 80-year-old uncle, who lives with us, seems to need more
attention from me every day as his memory gets worse and
worse. Since I already have to see that he takes several
medications on schedule, can I just add ginkgo to them?*

How safe it would be for your aged uncle to take ginkgo depends on what
his other medical problems are. If he falls into any of the categories listed

on page 174, you should consult with his doctor before adding ginkgo to his medication regimen. Note that we recommend that anyone who has multiple medical problems that require regular follow-up, with or without medication, should not take ginkgo without a doctor's supervision. Information from clinical studies as well as our clinical experience combines to indicate that ginkgo is generally well tolerated in otherwise healthy elderly people with dementia and may at least slow the progression of memory loss.

I'm 45. Should I start taking ginkgo to prevent memory loss or circulatory problems?

No studies to date show that ginkgo can prevent memory loss or circulatory problems. However, given ginkgo's wide range of therapeutic activity on various parts of the body and its antioxidant properties, coupled with its good tolerability and safety, it is very likely that the herb may have more long-range benefits. As we note on page 183, we have little information at this time on the extended long-term effects of ginkgo, but so far the herb has a good safety profile. Therefore, you may benefit from continued use of ginkgo. Start at 60 mg twice per day; consider increasing to 120 mg twice per day if ineffective after four to eight weeks. Further studies need to be conducted to explore ginkgo's prophylactic potential. Even if it cannot prevent memory loss, if it slows degeneration of cognitive functions it would be worth taking.

My child has school difficulties, trouble concentrating in class and at home. Would ginkgo be an appropriate choice for her?

The dosing guidelines on page 185 apply to adults 18 years of age or older. To date, systematic studies of ginkgo in children, if conducted, have not been published. Ginkgo seeds have been used as a part of TCM for all age groups over the centuries in China. They are reportedly safe in small quantities but highly toxic, causing seizures and loss of consciousness, in larger doses. While ginkgo extract has been used in children in some cultures, there is no scientific data to support its efficacy, and there are no clear indications for its use at this time. Given ginkgo's wide range of pharmacological activity and safety margin in adults, it seems plausible that ginkgo could exhibit similar activity in children. However, further study is warranted, and we therefore cannot recommend ginkgo use in children at this time.

*My best friend says he's improved his memory a thousandfold
with ginkgo. Exaggeration aside, can I expect the same effect
he's getting?*

Ginkgo does not work for everyone. Some people note a variety of improvements, such as enhanced alertness, memory, and concentration; increased energy; better sexual functioning; and improvement in general
well-being or other benefits. Others may observe only one or two changes,
while still others may not note a thing. Unfortunately, at this time, we cannot predict who will or will not have a favorable response. However, given
its range of potential benefits and good tolerability and safety, it is very reasonable to go ahead and give it a try.

*My 70-year-old grandmother has started to show signs of memory
loss, confusion, and inability to concentrate over the last few
weeks. My mother is planning to take her to the doctor for a
whole battery of tests to make sure nothing serious is wrong. I say
she's just showing the inevitable signs of aging and my mother
should just give her some ginkgo along with her vitamin in the
morning. Who's right?*

Your mother is! It's always possible that ginkgo could ease symptoms enough
to make them tolerable, thereby preventing a diagnosis of some other medical
condition that should be treated. However, the cognitive decline that occurs
with dementia in the elderly is usually gradual, with deterioration observed
over several years, not over weeks as demonstrated here. In such instances in
otherwise healthy adults, it is reasonable to consider a trial of ginkgo. If cognitive function improves or does not change, it is possible that ginkgo is helping, either through improvement or in staving off further deterioration. If the
condition worsens despite the use of ginkgo, it may just be the sad and unfor-
tunate natural course of the dementing process.

Deterioration, particularly rapid changes over days, weeks, and even
months, however, suggest that there is another process at work, one that
may be amenable to treatment. Conditions that can manifest in mental status changes and to which the elderly can be particularly susceptible include
the following:

- Dehydration
- Metabolic problems (e.g., low sodium, low blood sugar)

- Infections
- Brain lesions (e.g., strokes, cancer, trauma from head injury)
- Depression
- Heart, lung, liver, or kidney problems
- Impaired blood flow to the head
- Medication side effects and interactions

So a person who seems to suffer further decline while taking ginkgo should stop taking the herb and see his or her physician for further evaluation.

I've been diagnosed with dysthymia, and since I've had the condition my memory seems spotty. Would ginkgo help me?

It's often very difficult to determine if cognitive difficulties are related to depression or other emotional problems, such as anxiety, or if they are a separate problem altogether. This is a particularly challenging distinction to make in the elderly. If the problems are related to a primary anxiety or a mood problem, the deficits should improve with the treatment of the emotional disturbance. We do not know if ginkgo would provide extra benefit here, but it is possible, especially since ginkgo may have effects on certain brain chemicals. At this point, however, it is too early to tell. In cases where the cognitive deficits are related to a primary dementing process, ginkgo may be worth a trial.

You didn't mention if you were receiving treatment for your depression and, if so, what type of therapy and how effective it has been. If you're already inclined toward herbal medicine, you might consider St. John's wort for mild depression if you haven't already tried it (see Chapter 1). Talk to your doctor about this.

⚘ HOW GINKGO WORKS

Ginkgo biloba leaves contain a variety of chemical constituents (see Table 13). Among these, the medically active components are the flavone glycosides, bioflavonoids, and terpene lactones. Flavone glycosides and bioflavonoids are types of flavonoids, chemical compounds commonly found in many plants. The terpenoid constituents, ginkgolide A, B, C, J, and M and bilobalide, however, are characteristic of ginkgo alone.

Table 13. Chemical Constituents of Ginkgo Biloba Leaves

Flavonoids
    Flavonols, flavonol glycosides (quercetin, isorhamnetin, kaempferol)
    Biflavones
Terpenoids
    Diterpenes: ginkgolide A, B, C, J, M
    Sesquiterpene: bilobalide
Organic acids (e.g., ginkgolic acids)
Polyprenols
Other (e.g., waxes, steroids, sugars, proanthoccyanidins)

Note. Data from *Herbal PDR* (1998) and van Beek et al. (1998).

Flavonoids: Ginkgo's Free Radical Scavengers

Flavonoids are substances found in a variety of plants and fruits, particularly citrus fruits. They occur in plants as pigments in flowers and in fruits,
but their precise biological role in plants remains unknown. In humans,
they have several important functions in maintaining healthy cells and tissues. They are antioxidants and play an important role in the prevention of
tissue damage related to toxic oxygen free radicals (see box on facing page).
Flavonoids also help to keep cell membranes healthy by working to maintain their integrity and permeability. This is done by protecting cell membranes against the breakdown of arachidonic acid, an unsaturated fatty
acid, which is an important constituent of cell walls.

    As antioxidants, flavonoids clean up the circulating free radicals and
are thus called "free radical scavengers." In *Ginkgo biloba*, there are three
major flavone glycosides—isorhamnetin, quercetin, and kaempferol—the
last of which is unique to ginkgo. Some evidence suggests that ginkgo's
flavone glycosides may be even more effective antioxidants than either vitamin E or beta-carotene.

Bioflavonoids: Blood Vessel Fortifiers

The other clinically important flavonoids in ginkgo, the bioflavonoids,
play a more direct role in protecting blood vessels. These constituents help
to strengthen the walls of capillaries, the smallest blood vessels. Capillaries
are the sites of the interchange of various substances between blood and tissues, and in this capacity they deliver oxygen and other nutrients to tissues

while removing waste products to be carried away for excretion. These tiny blood vessels can become weak and leaky, due to injury and inflammation or to the effects of some medications such as certain types of steroids. This weakening leads to the inappropriate seepage of blood cells and other proteins out of the vessels and into the local surrounding tissues, causing tissue injury. The bioflavonoids in ginkgo help to prevent this from happening by strengthening the vessel walls and making them more resilient to trauma.

A Case for Not Freeing the Radicals

Free radicals (or "radicals") are atoms and molecules that are missing an electron, which renders them highly unstable and reactive. They may be naturally occurring in the body through normal processes, such as those produced by white blood cells in fighting invading microorganisms, and thus have a protective role. Free radicals are also generated in certain disease states and can be absorbed into the body through a variety of exposures, such as inhaling toxins (including some pollutants), ingesting harmful foods (including some fats), and being exposed to radiation, including sunlight, radiation therapy, and nuclear emissions. In such cases, radicals can be quite harmful, causing a cascade of events whereby cells are damaged, tissues break down, and ultimately cells die. In some cases, free radicals generate a chain reaction and cause more damage. One particular target for free radicals are phospholipids, essential constituents of cell membranes and nerve cells (including those in the brain). Free radical injury has been implicated in a variety of disease states including AD, heart disease, cancer, and the inflammation producing arthritic changes, as well as in the physiological changes associated with aging.

To achieve stability, free radicals interact with other electronically intact atoms and molecules, such as normal cells in the body, by removing one of their electrons. While the radical is now stable and happy, it has left behind a cell that is injured and potentially unstable itself. When multiple cells are injured in this fashion, it can lead to tissue and organ damage and serious consequences.

These radicals are neutralized by substances called *free radical scavengers* or *antioxidants*. Antioxidants work by donating electrons to free radicals, thereby rendering them neutralized and stable. We have naturally occurring antioxidants in our systems, such as an enzyme called *superoxide dismutase*. A number of popular supplements also have antioxidant activity, including vitamins A, C, and E, beta-carotene, and *Ginkgo biloba*. Antioxidant properties are also found in several foods, notably blueberries and strawberries.

Terpene Lactones: Blood Clot Regulators

The terpenoid constituents are the ginkgolides and bilobalides. The first ginkoglides were initially isolated in a ginkgo extract back in the 1930s. Several decades later scientists discovered their complex and characteristic cagelike chemical structure. To date, five ginkgolides have been identified: A, B, C, J, and M. Discovered in the 1960s, the bilobalides are less complicated structurally. The unique structure of the ginkgolides is almost impossible to reproduce; attempts to synthesize these molecules in the laboratory have resulted in repeated failures. Therefore, the only source of ginkgolides at this time remains nature.

The terpene lactones help to reduce the adhesion of platelets, the blood cells responsible for clotting and that help to stop bleeding when we are cut. Platelets have a tendency to want to stick together, particularly in the presence of a substance called *platelet activating factor* (PAF). PAF, produced by a variety of different blood cells, is a natural mediator of inflammation (e.g., in response to trauma or the presence of foreign organisms), platelet aggregation, and constriction of blood vessels. By sticking together, platelets form blood clots. At times when we are injured and bleeding, clot formation is a good thing. However, clots can also form *within* our blood vessels, with serious consequences if they obstruct the free flow of blood with its supply of nutrients. When this happens in the very small vessels in the brain and heart, parts of these vital organs are deprived of oxygen, glucose, and other nutrients, leading to cell injury and often cell death, and can result in organ malfunction.

By antagonizing the effects of PAF, ginkgolides A, B, and C, but particularly B, prevent the attachment of PAF to receptors on platelet cell membranes and thereby reduce platelet "stickiness." This is very likely one mechanism by which ginkgo improves circulation, keeping blood flowing to the brain and other vital tissues and organs.

Terpenoids may also play a role in the protection of nerve cells. When blood flow to an area is compromised (usually due to obstruction by a clot or a vessel narrowing from vasoconstriction or by buildup of atherosclerotic plaques and other debris), insufficient nutrients are delivered to tissues. This state of deprivation can result in tissue injury called *ischemia*. Ginkgolides A and B and bilobalide have been shown to protect nerve cells in brains subjected to periods of ischemia. In this way, ginkgo may help to reduce nerve cell damage following injuries such as small strokes, or transient ischemic attacks (TIAs).

Ginkgo's constituents exert their effects in several ways when in the proper balance, acting simultaneously in concert, in combination, and synergistically. To achieve these effects, ginkgo extracts should be standardized on their flavone glycoside and terpene lactone content. The German Commission E recommends that extracts contain 22 to 27 percent flavone glycosides (average 24 percent) and 5 to 7 percent terpene lactones (average 6 percent).

From Chemicals to Remedies

As you can guess from its mechanisms of action, ginkgo has a range of pharmacological activities. Let's look more closely at how ginkgo protects vessels and tissues and enhances cognitive function.

Blood vessels, the tissues they supply, and nerves are protected by ginkgo in a number of different ways—some of them already discussed. Ginkgo helps to modulate blood vessel tone, relaxing vessels in spasm while increasing the tone of abnormally relaxed vessels. Remarkably, and fortunately, ginkgo does not seem to affect vessels that are contracting or dilating in response to normal physiological changes. Ginkgo also helps to maintain the integrity of vessel walls and their permeability, allowing some substances to pass through directly while preventing leakage or the unwanted entry of others. This is a particularly important function at the level of the capillaries, where oxygen and other nutrients are exchanged for cell waste by-products. It is also important in reducing edema, or swelling, which can occur with leakage of substances out of vessels or nerves into surrounding areas, leading to tissue injury. Finally, as discussed earlier, ginkgo protects vessels, tissues, and nerves by inhibiting platelet aggregation and clot formation and by reducing injury caused by ischemic insults.

Ginkgo enhances cognitive functioning in several ways, effects that may in part be related to the antioxidant properties of the ginkgo flavonoids. It enhances the release of specific neurochemicals that affect nervous system function (e.g., catecholamines and other neurotransmitters), while inhibiting the reuptake of others. Ginkgo also inhibits certain enzymes (catechol-O-methyl transferase, monoamine oxidase, and certain proteases) that are involved in the breakdown of a number of neurochemicals that affect brain regions associated with behavior and mentation. It also protects endothelial derived relaxing factor (EDRF; a substance released from within blood vessel walls that causes vessels to relax or dilate as needed and that is now known to be nitric oxide) from damage by free radicals.

These effects have been observed at a variety of cellular levels and on multiple organ systems. In its ginkgo monograph, the German Commission E lists the following actions for ginkgo extract:

- Increases tissue tolerance to oxygen deprivation, especially in the brain.
- Increases blood flow, especially in the microcirculation (e.g., the capillaries, where substances are interchanged on a molecular level between the blood and tissues).
- Enhances the properties of blood that facilitate blood flow.
- Inhibits the development of brain swelling (or edema) following trauma or toxic injury and hastens its resolution.
- In the eye, reduces retinal swelling and cellular lesions.
- Facilitates compensation in equilibrium disturbances, especially conditions related to microcirculatory problems.
- Improves memory performance and learning capacity.
- Prevents cell and tissue damage by scavenging and inactivating toxic oxygen-derived free radicals.
- Inhibits the development of age-related decreases in specific neurochemical receptors that are sites of attachment in the brain for certain chemicals (muscarinergic, cholinoceptors, and $\alpha2$-adrenoceptors).
- Promotes uptake of a specific neurochemical, choline, involved in the production of phospholipids in the hippocampus, a brain region involved in memory.
- Inhibits platelet aggregation and clot formation by antagonizing platelet activating factor.
- Protects nerve cells from ischemic injury during periods of insufficient blood flow.
- A number of other biological effects have been reported but are less well characterized, including inhibition of monoamine oxidase A and B and promotion of glucose uptake and utilization. Further investigation is needed before any conclusions can be drawn about ginkgo's clinical utility in these areas, but at this time we are unaware of any particular studies under way.

As you can see, ginkgo is a truly unique compound, really unlike any other natural or synthetic product.

Safety Issues

It's hard to believe that a single herb could offer so many health benefits at so little cost to the body. But adverse effects are rare with the standardized ginkgo extract. In their compendium of monographs, the German Commission E notes rare incidence of stomach or intestinal upset (less than 1 percent in clinical studies), headaches, or allergic skin reaction. Other reported side effects have included mild transient dizziness. No particular constituent has been found to be associated with these effects.

Animal studies of both the acute and chronic effects of ginkgo have repeatedly demonstrated a wide margin of safety for ginkgo extract. Furthermore, in these studies, ginkgo was not associated with teratogenic or mutagenic effects.

While extract from the dried leaves is quite safe, adverse effects have been reported with use of other parts of the plant. Direct skin contact with the fresh pulp of ginkgo fruit frequently results in an allergic contact dermatitis, similar to that seen with allergic reactions to poison ivy. Ingestion of the fresh pulp can also produce an allergic reaction, causing severe irritation and inflammation from one end of the gastrointestinal tract to the other.

Raw ginkgo nuts, another name for ginkgo seeds, have long been associated with toxic reactions in humans and insects, attributed in part to the seed's ginkgolic acid content. In fact, the shells of the nuts were used in ancient China and Japan as an insecticide. By boiling the nuts, the toxins were neutralized and the seeds were considered acceptable for human consumption. Today, ginkgo nuts are available only in the East. While steeped in the traditions of TCM, use of unspecified excessive amounts of these seeds has been associated with seizures, loss of consciousness, and even death, with particular sensitivity observed in children.

While believed to be quite safe, the *Ginkgo biloba* leaf and seed do contain some toxic elements that have been associated with allergic reactions. These responses are exceedingly rare today, as a result of the processes of extract standardization and with the knowledge of how the plant parts should be safely handled. This should not be an issue for consumers who buy standardized products. Just don't pick a fruit off a tree on the streets of New York, handle the fresh pulp of the fruits, or eat the seeds.

Though we don't have as much information about long-term use of ginkgo, in a controlled clinical study of ginkgo in elderly adults with dementia, adverse effects observed did not differ between subjects receiving ginkgo and those receiving a placebo after 52 weeks of treatment (Le Bars et al., 1997). While we do not have information from controlled studies extending beyond one year, anecdotal evidence indicates no adverse effects with long-term use. Furthermore, tolerance, dependence, and/or withdrawal (physiological or psychological) symptoms have not been reported with ginkgo, and we would not expect them to be problems.

Interactions, a common issue with all medications, herbal and pharmaceutical, also seem to be a much lesser concern with ginkgo. The German Commission E, for one, makes no cautions about use or interactions with other drugs. However, as we said earlier, those taking blood thinners (anticoagulants or antithrombotics), such as coumadin, should not take ginkgo, nor should alcoholics with severe liver disease, because they can develop a deficiency in vitamin K, which leads to clotting problems.

Interestingly, considering that ginkgo can ease one of the side effects of SSRIs, some caution should be exercised by people taking SSRIs. There is a small but growing body of evidence from animal and human studies showing that SSRIs have some degree of PAF inhibition and could theoretically contribute to bleeding problems in those taking ginkgo. This is potentially an important point given the widespread and growing prescription of SSRIs. So until further information is available, consumers should be alert to this potential problem and exercise caution if using ginkgo, perhaps considering lower doses of both—but don't do this without checking with your doctor first!

Over the last few years, as the use of ginkgo has continued to spread, several case reports have been published describing the development of intracranial (i.e., within the head) bleeding with chronic ginkgo use: one case of bleeding in the eye, one brain hemorrhage, and two cases of bleeding in the space between the skull and the brain. In two of the cases the patients were also taking either aspirin or a blood thinner. These reports did not prove that ginkgo caused or even contributed to the hemorrhages. Nonetheless, with the knowledge that we have of ginkgo's antiplatelet and anticlotting effects, until further study, the herb should not be used if you are taking blood thinners; if you use aspirin daily, talk with your doctor first. If you have any other risk factors for developing a hemorrhagic stroke (high blood pressure, diabetes, heavy alcohol use, cigarette smoking), you should not use ginkgo without your physician's approval.

There are no known dangers in overdose. In fact, in general ginkgo has a wide margin for safety. While there have been a handful of case reports of serious events in people taking ginkgo (as noted above), these have been very rare—far less frequent than serious events with many prescription medications. It is very important, however, always to let your doctor know when you are taking herbs or other dietary supplements, as well as other as-needed over-the-counter medications of any type.

Is it safe to take ginkgo and drink alcoholic beverages?

No problems are known with concurrent alcohol use. One concern we have, however, is related to the increased risks of falls and head injury in people who drink heavily. People may not recall such falls and injuries be-cause of intoxication and they may go unnoticed by others if there is no ob-vious and visible injury. Nonetheless, these injuries can involve internal bleeding (of the head in particular with head injury)—or external bleeding for that matter. Hypothetically, given one of ginkgo's mechanisms of ac-tion, it is possible that bleeding problems could occur. So, if we knew that a patient tended to binge on alcohol or suffered from chronic alcoholism, we would not recommend ginkgo.

✒ HOW TO USE GINKGO

How Much Ginkgo to Take and When

Standardized ginkgo extract comes in 40-mg, 60-mg, 80-mg, and 120-mg tablets, though the 60-mg tablets are the most common. Dose ranges are between 120 and 240 mg of extract per day taken in divided doses. So with the 60-mg tablets, this translates into anywhere from one to two tablets twice a day. Practitioners of TCM administer ginkgo in a tea infu-sion, using anywhere from three to six grams of crude, dried leaves per day.

Dosage recommendations may vary somewhat among products. While most standardized products contain dose units of 60 mg, we found a wide range of recommendations in our recent survey of herbal product brands (see Table 14). Of the standardized products surveyed and listing milligram dosages (17 out of 20), doses ranged from 40 mg to 450 mg per tablet, with recommendations for taking anywhere from a minimum of one tablet (40 mg) to a maximum of six tablets (433 mg). This translates into doses from 40 mg to over 2,400 mg per day. (We should note that the products listing doses of 400 to 450 mg were not just listing the

Table 14. Comparisons of Different Brands of Ginkgo Available in Three Different Retail Stores (November 1998)

Store	Brand	Dose/pill	Pills/day	Standardized	Other ingredients	Expiration date	Cost/day
1	A	400 mg	2–6 as needed	No	Yes (2)	Yes	$0.22–0.66
	B	450 mg	3 as needed	Yes	No	Yes	$0.48
2	C	433 mg	6	Yes	Yes (3)	Yes	$0.42
	D	450 mg	3	Yes	No	Yes	$0.30
	E	450 mg	3	Yes	Yes (2)	Yes	$0.30
	F	450 mg	3	Yes	No	Yes	$0.36
	G	400 mg	3	Yes	No	Yes	$0.42
	H	40 mg	?	Yes	No	Yes	—[a]
	I	40 mg	3	Yes	No	Yes	$0.33
	J	60 mg	2–4	Yes	No	Yes	$0.84–1.68
3	K	?	120–160 drops	No	No	No	—[a]
	L	40 mg	3	Yes	No	Yes	1.08
	M	120 mg	1	Yes	No	No	$0.37
	N	40 mg	1–3	Yes	No	No	$0.15–0.45
	O	40 mg	3	Yes	No	No	$0.75
	P	80 mg	3	Yes	Yes (1)	No	$0.99
	Q	60 mg	1–3	Yes	No	No	$0.23–0.69
	R	60 mg	1 or more	Yes	No	Yes	$0.27 or
	S	60 mg	2	Yes	Yes (2)	Yes	$0.72
	T	?	2–9	Yes	No	No	$0.48–1.44

Note. ?, no dose specified.
[a]Unable to determine cost per day with information available.

186

ginkgo content, and several were combination products.) The majority of products recommended taking 120 to 240 mg per day. You don't need to take it with food, but it can be helpful to take it with meals just for the sake of convenience.

The doses used in most of the clinical studies and found to be effective were between 120 mg and 180 mg per day. Some studies suggest that higher doses of 240 mg per day are needed in more severe cases of dementia. We generally recommend starting with anywhere from 120 to 180 mg per day and giving this dosage a good trial of 8 to 10 weeks. Increase to 240 mg per day if you don't see improvements. For sexual dysfunction related to antidepressant medication, we recommend moving to the high end of the dose scale, 240 mg per day. It is important to take ginkgo daily to benefit from its full effects. It does not seem to have the same activity and confer the same benefits when taken sporadically.

As with all things, U.S. manufacturers always seem keen to come out with "new and improved" products. In the case of ginkgo, extended-release preparations have recently been appearing in the stores. We are not aware of any clinical studies supporting the use of these formulations. Are they truly time-released products? If so, how do they work (pharmacokinetically and pharmacologically)? Putting an enteric coating on the tablets does not necessarily mean that the pharmacokinetic and pharmacodynamic properties of the product are consistent with a timed release. Are they at least as good as the ginkgo formulations that are currently available? Are there any other safety concerns? They will almost invariably cost more than immediate-release tablets, presumably because of the expense of developing the extended-release technology. At this point in time, we would recommend caution in using these new products. Stick with what seems to work. If they work, sound scientific information supporting their use should be just around the corner!

Brand Choices

Do ginkgo products vary in potency depending on brand? Is there a way to tell?

This should not be an issue with standardized extracts. As with other herbs, there is seasonal variation in the content of the leaves: the highest flavone glycoside content is found in fresh leaves harvested in May. Great care is taken to keep the leaves dry after collection, to prevent moisture-related fermentation.

The extraction process is conducted in a standardized fashion. The leaves are mixed with solvents to produce a primary crude extract with an herb:extract ratio of roughly 4:1. This crude product undergoes further processing and concentration to remove unwanted products and yield a much more potent extract. To meet manufacturing specifications and quality control standards set by the German Commission E, a ginkgo product must have an herb:extract ratio of between 35:1 and 67:1 (average 50:1) and have undergone extraction with an acetone–water mixture and further purification without the addition of other constituents. Two extracts that have met these standards and are used in drug manufacture in Germany (and in some U.S. products) are EGb 761 and LI 1370.

Products should be stored in a manner that protects them from light and moisture.

If there's no danger of overdose and no side effects, won't I stand a better chance of improving the more ginkgo I take?

As with almost everything, more is not always better. The information we have on the safety and effectiveness of ginkgo stems from scientific research and clinical experience. Based on both of these, we recommend doses of up to 240 mg per day. Sure, higher doses have been used in some studies for specific indications, but only in a handful of people. It is possible that at higher does there may be significant side effects that are not experienced at the lower doses. So the use of higher doses across the board is an issue that needs further study. The jury is still out on this one.

Is there a chance that side effects will vary among brands?

This is unlikely with standardized ginkgo extracts. But remember that everyone is different in their sensitivities to medications and herbs. Someone could have different side effects with different brands, but most likely only if they are not standardized products. The place to be alert for variation in side effects is in the use of combination products. At this time, however, there is no evidence to support the use of products containing ginkgo and other herbs. So if you stick with the standardized single ginkgo preparations, you should be fine.

Is It Working?

As with other medications and dietary supplements, responses vary from one person to the next. Some users note benefits in just a few weeks, but others take a bit longer to see a positive response. Improvement will often occur after eight to 12 weeks of treatment, though changes may be subtle at first and take longer in the case of dementia. If after this time you have not had any effects and are taking 120 mg per day, try increasing the dose, up to 180 mg per day, and, if needed, to 240 mg per day. If after eight weeks or so at the full dose you have not noticed an appreciable effect, it is probably time to consider switching brands.

Unfortunately, because ginkgo has the potential to affect such a variety of organ systems, self-tests of effectiveness are impractical. While rating scales have been developed to measure severity of cognitive impairment, these tap into a lot more than just memory and concentration, and are not particularly useful outside of the doctor's office or the research lab. Any improvement you gain will generally be quite subjective.

Ginkgo's popularity is due in part to its longevity (remember, it has been called "a living fossil"); products that work tend to stick around, and their benefits spread by word of mouth. A lot can be spread by word of mouth in 200 million years. In Europe, particularly in Germany and France, ginkgo's popularity is a testament to its effectiveness and safety. Whether it works for you is for you to judge.

I like the extra sharpness I have now that I'm taking ginkgo. Is there any reason not to keep taking it indefinitely, like any other dietary supplements such as vitamins?

At this time, there are no contraindications to the long-term use of ginkgo. It should be noted, however, that safety information from controlled clinical studies is limited to one year. Keep this caution in mind if you plan to use ginkgo for a longer period of time.

It is also unclear how long ginkgo's effects are observed: Do you get the effects only when taking it, or do changes persist for some time after discontinuation of the herb? There is some evidence in favor of the latter hypothesis. For example, recalling the effects of ginkgo in people exposed to nuclear radiation following the Soviet Chernobyl nuclear disaster in 1986, after treatment for two months, the positive effects of ginkgo were observed for up 10 months following treatment discontinuation in some people. A similar effect may be observed with other clinical applications; however, additional research is needed to substantiate these effects. We are not aware of any such ongoing studies at this time.

I'm trying to save money wherever I can, since I just lost my job unexpectedly. What will happen if I stop taking ginkgo all at once? Any rebound effect?

Abrupt discontinuation of Ginkgo biloba is believed to be safe. Ginkgo is not associated with physiological dependence, tolerance, or withdrawal. So if you suddenly stop taking your ginkgo, you should not experience any adverse effects. Remember, though, that if you are taking a combination product containing ginkgo and other herbs, it is possible that you could have some discomfort. This would be related to discontinuation of the other herbs in the preparation, however.

What Lies Ahead?

Ginkgo is truly nature's resilient wonder. In some ways it seems to possess the ability to confer this resilience on those who use it. With the information we have to date, the future seems ripe for further investigation into this fascinating herb. Can ginkgo help us live longer, healthier lives? While we cannot yet answer this question, we can identify a number of promising areas in need of further study:

- Effectiveness and safety in long-term daily use and at higher doses
- Use in performance enhancement, such as when studying for and taking a test
- Effectiveness compared to other treatments currently being used for dementia (as examined through controlled studies)
- Use in early intervention for those at risk for and in the early stages of dementia (the key here is finding a way to identify members of these groups early and to determine whether treatment is helpful when instituted at that time)
- Effects in combating SSRI-induced and other medication-associated and medically related forms of sexual dysfunction (e.g., from hyper-

tension, heart disease, diabetes, and primary sexual dysfunction that is not related to another medical condition or medication)

- Use as a prophylactic in staving off certain heart problems—is it cardioprotective or "heart healthy," as we have found aspirin to be, and should it be taken daily?
- Safety in children—and with what benefit in children?

ESSENTIAL FACTS ABOUT GINKGO	
Main Uses	Slowing of age-related cognitive decline such as memory deficits, possibly improvement of mental performance in those with normal memory capacity
Other Reported Uses	Treatment for intermittent claudication, tinnitus, vertigo, altitude sickness, asthma, and antidepressant-induced sexual dysfunction; antioxidant; promotes blood circulation; some reversal of age-related decline in vision and other senses; antioxidant protection from radiation exposure
When Not to Use This Herb	While taking anticoagulants (blood thinners); bleeding or clotting disorders or serious liver disease; when pregnant, trying to conceive, or breastfeeding; taking aspirin daily (talk with your doctor first)
Side Effects	Stomach or intestinal upset, headaches, allergic skin reaction, mild transient dizziness—all rare
When to Expect Positive Effects	After 2 to 12 weeks of use; full effect usually within 8 to 12 weeks
Common Preparation Forms	Tablets, liquid, dried leaves for brewing tea
Average Effective Daily Dosage	120 to 240 mg standardized extract, taken in divided doses one to three times a day

4

Valerian

Nature's Sandman

When we are tired, we are attacked by ideas we conquered
long ago.
                            —FRIEDRICH WILHELM NIETZSCHE

Shakespeare dubbed it "nature's soft nurse."
Coleridge called it "a gentle thing, beloved
from pole to pole." The subject was sleep, a natural function that should
absorb perhaps eight hours of every adult's day but eludes up to a third of
the population at some point in life. Without a good night's sleep, we spend
our waking hours feeling edgy and impatient, spacy and distracted, tired,
inefficient, and overwhelmed by the demands of life. No wonder we seek
help both with falling asleep and with staying asleep.

Unfortunately, much of what the pharmacist and the drugstore shelves
offer us doesn't do the trick. Sleep is a complicated function, and not all
sleep aids are effective for all people. When they do work, their cost may be
too high: We sleep, but we feel drugged, groggy, or hungover the next day.
If we keep taking them, we may find our sleep aids habit-forming, such that
we become unable to sleep without them or need more and more to fall
asleep over time. Taking too much of a sleep aid or combining a sleep aid
with alcohol or other medications can be dangerous—even fatal.

Today's health food stores offer a number of natural, gentle alternatives to prescription sleep aids, from classic chamomile tea, to multiherb

concoctions of everything from passionflower to hops, to the widely publicized melatonin. But what tops many shopping lists is valerian, a perennial herb whose medicinal qualities, notably sleep assistance, have been well documented for at least 2,000 years. In 1998 valerian was number 12 on the U.S. list of top-selling herbs, and with good reason: of all the herbal remedies on the market today, valerian has been used most widely to promote sleep, and the body of scientific literature supporting its use as a sleep aid is fairly substantial.

Still, we don't know everything we'd like to know about this herbal remedy. Is it the best natural sleep aid for most people? How long can one take it safely? Is it most effective on its own or in combination with other soporific herbs? How does one choose among the numerous valerian products available on the shelves today?

What's in a Name?

Exactly where the name *valerian* originated is unknown, but clearly those who dubbed it believed it had powerful benefits. *Valerian* is derived from the Latin *valere*, meaning health or well-being, or courage, as in *valor*.

Beware of confusing similar-named herbs with valerian. American valerian (lady's slipper or pink lady's slipper), garden heliotrope, Greek valerian (Jacob's ladder), and life roots (false valerian) are not *Valeriana* species and do not possess the properties of valerian.

🌿 WHAT VALERIAN DOES

Valerian is best known as a sleep aid. It's shelved with the other sleep aids that you're likely to find in any health food store. According to the German Commission E Monographs and the American *Herbal PDR*, *Valeriana officinalis*—the species, among 200, of the genus *Valeriana* most commonly used in herbal medicine—can be used to treat restlessness and sleeping disorders based on nervous conditions. The fact that the herb relaxes people so they can sleep may explain why valerian could also be a good over-the-counter remedy for those suffering from stress and tension. Though we haven't studied its anxiety-reducing effects systematically, a number of studies of valerian for sleep have shown that it improves anxiety, mood, and general well-being along with insomnia. Also, people subjected to mild stress conditions, such as driving in traffic or having to perform on a test or other task, have reported that valerian reduced their anxiety. Moreover, valerian has been used in Europe for the last 100 years to treat menopausal nervous anxiety, hysteria, nervous irritability, and even shell shock.

We often recommend valerian to our patients for sleep problems and mild anxiety because the evidence of its effectiveness and safety in treating these troubles is fairly strong. But like most other traditional herbal medicines, it has been used over the centuries to treat a wide variety of diseases and disorders, to alleviate all kinds of aches and pains, and even to bestow special power or fortune. According to folklore, valerian will not only give you a good night's rest, but also supply you with an endless queue of ardent lovers if you are a young woman who carries a sprig around with you, or keep you and your spouse from bickering if you hang a sprig in your home. It could increase your psychic perception, protect you from thunder and lightning, enhance your powers of witchcraft, or arm you against spells cast by others. It is said to attract cats, especially male cats, and bring them to a state of ecstasy. Apparently it excites rats too; some say it was valerian in his pocket, not his musical prowess, that enabled the Pied Piper to charm the rats of Hamelin. The less fanciful uses that valerian has enjoyed at other times, in other places, are listed in the box below. As time goes on, we expect research to tell us more about valerian's powers in these areas.

An Adaptable Herb: Valerian across the World and through the Ages

- Historically, valerian has been reported to have hypnotic (sleep-inducing), sedative (relaxing), antispasmodic (muscle-spasm-reducing), mild analgesic (pain-relieving), carminative (gas-relieving), and hypotensive (blood-pressure-lowering) properties.
- Valerian has been used to treat hysterical states, nervous excitability, insomnia, hypochondriasis, migraine, cramps, intestinal colic, rheumatic pains, and pain associated with the menstrual cycle.
- In India, the variety *Nardostachys jatamansi* DC. Mem. is used to treat epilepsy, hysteria, other convulsive ailments, palpitations of the

heart, consumption, diseases of the eye, itch, boils, swellings, diseases of the head, and hiccough. In contrast, *Valeriana wallichii* DC. Mem. is used as an ingredient in a snake bite remedy, as well as in the treatment of liver, kidney, and spleen disorders.

- Similar uses have been reported with a variety of other species in Chinese medicine, where valerian has also been used for chronic backache, numbness due to rheumatic conditions, colds, menstrual difficulties, bruises, and sores.
- Valerian is also used for a number of nonmedicinal purposes: in cosmetics, in topical applications, and as a food source. In some cultures, valerian is used in perfume and herbal baths and as a mild tea in facial washes. As an alcohol extract, valerian has been used to treat dandruff, acne, skin rashes, and other sores. As a food source, leaves of the valerian plant have been used in salad in place of lettuce or spinach.
- In A.D. 40–80, Dioscorides recommended several species of *Valeriana* (phu) for digestive problems, nausea, liver problems, and urinary tract disorders.
- The ancient Greek physician and pharmacist Galen (A.D. 129–ca. 199) made the first allusions to valerian's sedative qualities.
- In the 16th and 17th centuries, valerian was reported to be effective in treating epilepsy.
- In the 18th century valerian came into common use as a sedative and in treating a variety of nervous disorders. Reported uses of valerian at this time included the treatment of rheumatism, low-grade fevers, hysteria, epilepsy, menopausal nervous anxiety, and nervous irritability attributable to an "enfeebled cerebral circulation." It was also used as an analgesic and an aphrodisiac.
- During World War I, tincture of valerian was used as a tranquilizer to treat soldiers suffering from shell shock.
- Valerian has been included in a number of official pharmacological texts in the United States over the years, including the *United States Pharmacopoeia* (USP) from 1821 to 1936 and the *United States National Formulary* until 1946.
- Valerian today is listed in the pharmacopoeias of Austria, Brazil, Czechoslovakia, Egypt, France, Germany, Great Britain, Greece, Hungary, Italy, the Netherlands, Norway, Romania, Russia, Switzerland, and Yugoslavia. In the 1983 version of the *British Herbal Pharmacopoeia*, valerian is described as a sedative, mild anodyne, hypnotic, spasmolytic, carminative, and hypotensive that is indicated for hysterical states, excitability, insomnia, hypochondriasis, migraine, cramp, and rheumatic pain.

Why Can't You Sleep?

People lose sleep for many different reasons, from bad sleep habits to stress and worry to medical or psychiatric illness. Sometimes insomnia lasts for only one night, sometimes for several, and sometimes it becomes a chronic problem. Some people need only make a few simple changes in lifestyle to get a good night's sleep night after night, some need more complicated behavioral techniques or psychotherapy, and some need medicine. What will work best for you depends largely on what is causing your lack of sleep.

The inability to get to sleep and/or to stay asleep for the time you expect is called *insomnia*. It's important to know that insomnia is a sleep complaint, not a disorder in and of itself (except in cases of primary insomnia in which the cause is unknown). My insomnia may be caused by a breathing problem known as sleep apnea, whereas yours might be the simple result of your insistence on eating a big bowl of chili with chopped onion and cheese right before climbing into bed. Your neighbor on one side may have trouble falling asleep because she does her vigorous workout right before retiring, mistakenly believing it will wear her out, while your neighbor on the other side may wake up at 3:00 every morning and find it impossible to get back to sleep because he suffers from depression. No wonder, then, that you can't call your doctor and expect over-the-phone treatment advice—or that you can't walk into a drugstore and grab the first "sleeping pill" you see on the shelf and expect it to solve your problem. First you need to find out why you can't sleep.

Sleep disorders fall into two categories, shown in Table 15. *Dyssomnias* are disorders in which you have trouble falling asleep or staying asleep or sleep excessively. They range from the unusual—such as sleep apnea, in which you partially wake up on and off throughout the night due to several seconds of interrupted breathing—to the temporary, such as jet lag, to the most common problem of all, loss of sleep due to lifestyle factors, particularly stress and poor sleep habits of various kinds. *Parasomnias* are disorders in which you are awakened or you don't progress normally from one sleep stage to the next. They include things like sleepwalking and bedwetting and also sleep disruptions caused by psychiatric and medical conditions.

Are you losing sleep because of elevated stress levels, because you have a food allergy, because you are alcoholic, because you sleepwalk, because you suffer from panic disorder, or for some other reason? If you eliminate excess stress from your life, cut out the offending food, or stop drinking, your insomnia may very well disappear on its own. If you suffer from panic

Table 15. Sleep Disorders

Dyssomnias (literally = "ill" or "bad" sleep)

Disorders of sleep and wakefulness.

Characterized by trouble initiating and maintaining sleep or by sleeping excessively.

Intrinsic disorders: originate with or are caused by some condition(s) in the body. Examples include narcolepsy, sleep apnea syndrome, restless legs syndrome, periodic limb movement disorder, primary insomnia.

Extrinsic disorders: the cause arises outside of the body. Examples include poor sleep hygiene, altitude insomnia, food allergy insomnia, disorders associated with alcohol or drug dependence.

Circadian rhythm disorders: irregularities of sleep that relate to mechanisms that regulate the 24-hour sleep–wake cycle. Examples include jet lag and shift work.

Parasomnias (literally = "besides" or "beyond" sleep)

Disorders of transition from one sleep stage to another, arousal, or partial arousal.

Examples include sleepwalking, sleep talking, nocturnal leg cramps, night terrors, nightmares, sleep paralysis, enuresis (i.e., bedwetting).

Sleep disorders associated with medical or psychiatric disorders

Not primarily sleep disorders, but are associated with sleep disturbance.

Associated with mental disorders: examples include mood disorders (e.g., depression, bipolar disorder), anxiety disorders (e.g., obsessive–compulsive disorder, posttraumatic stress disorder, panic disorder, generalized anxiety disorder, social anxiety disorder), psychoses, alcoholism.

Associated with neurological disorders: examples include dementia, parkinsonism.

Associated with other medical disorders: examples include chronic obstructive pulmonary disease (i.e., emphysema), sleep-related asthma, gastroesophageal reflux, peptic ulcer disease.

---

disorder or sleepwalking, whether your insomnia goes away may depend on the treatment you're receiving for the disorder that is causing it.

Insomnia is a common symptom of major depression and of a number of anxiety disorders (such as posttraumatic stress disorder and generalized anxiety disorder). Many different medical conditions, listed in Table 16, can also cause insomnia. So if you treat *only* your insomnia, you may be leaving any underlying condition undiagnosed and untreated. This can mean letting a harmful condition progress and allowing your daily functioning to continue to deteriorate despite the fact that you are sleeping better.

Table 16. Medical Conditions Associated with Sleep Disturbances

- Pain of any source
- Lung disorders
  - Chronic obstructive pulmonary disease (i.e., emphysema)
- Kidney disorders
  - Uremia (buildup of waste products in the bloodstream)
  - Urinary tract infection
- Endocrine disorders
  - Hyperthyroidism
  - Hypothyroidism
- Steroids and other medications
- Heart disorders
  - Nocturnal angina (chest pain that occurs at night at rest)
  - Orthopnea (awakening due to shortness of breath caused by impaired heart function)
- Dementia
- Delirium (due to infections, medication side effects or drug interactions)

When Should You Treat Insomnia?

Our sleep is very sensitive to the day-to-day events in our lives, as well as to our experiences over time. During periods of high productivity, we may actually need *less* sleep; yet, because such periods are generally also associated with more stress and anxiety, we may subjectively feel that we need *more* rest. Exercise and activity affect sleep, generally by reducing the time required to fall asleep and by promoting a deeper, longer period of rest.

If your insomnia is causing problems with your day-to-day functioning, has led to your use of stimulants such as caffeine or over-the-counter "pick-me-ups" just to stay awake, and/or does not resolve when you are in a more relaxing environment (e.g., on vacation or over the weekends), and it has continued for several weeks or months without any improvement, you should consult your primary care physician to see if the sleep problem may be masking a more significant condition that warrants medical attention.

If, on the other hand, your insomnia is a recent intruder in your life or it plagues you only occasionally and relatively briefly, you may not have to treat it at all. Insomnia may well go away without any active intervention from you. The determining factor in whether to treat or not to treat your insomnia is how debilitating it is. Some people can operate on half their usual sleep for days, while others feel "off" for several days if they get two hours' less sleep than normal for even one night. Insomnia typically causes these problems:

- Irritability and edginess
- Impatience with colleagues at the office, with friends, and with family members at home
- Poor concentration and inattentiveness
- Easily distracted by other things
- Low energy with easy fatigability
- Inefficiency and lower productivity
- Anxiety related to not getting things done
- Feeling more overwhelmed with day-to-day stresses and demands

As long as you find such effects tolerable, you can try to ride out your insomnia or take the least intrusive measures to counteract it, such as deep breathing or relaxation exercises to help you unwind and fall asleep. Be aware, however, that the longer insomnia persists, the more debilitating its adverse effects may become. A sleep-deprived truck driver, for example, may be more prone to accidents due to drifting off to sleep at the wheel.

We really don't know how long people can go without sleep without suffering irreversible consequences. For most people, *the time to treat insomnia is when it starts to make the days as miserable as the nights.* If you have reached that point, you have a number of treatment options.

Which Treatment Is Right for You?

Physician-Supervised Treatments

If you consult a doctor, the treatment choices available to you will fall into the categories of behavioral treatments, psychotherapy, drugs, and—less commonly—surgery or medical devices.

Behavioral treatments such as sleep restriction (restricting time spent in bed to sleeping), stimulus control (reinforcing the mental link between the bedroom and sleep), relaxation therapy, biofeedback, and chronotherapy (broadly defined as the coordination of treatment with a person's inherent biological rhythms) can not only help you recover from a bout of insomnia but also give you skills to fall back on should your insomnia return. But all these treatments require a significant investment of time from you. The same applies to psychotherapy, often used as an adjunct to behavioral or medicinal treatments in recognition of the fact that emotional disorders, such as depression and anxiety, often cause insomnia.

Interest in the effectiveness of nonmedication treatments for insomnia has been growing. In fact a study published in the *Journal of the American Medical Association* looked at behavioral versus medication treatments for late-life insomnia (Morin et al., 1999). The researchers compared four different treatments: cognitive-behavioral therapy (CBT; comprised of stimulus control, sleep restriction, sleep hygiene, and cognitive therapy), Restoril (a benzodiazepine), a combination of these two, and placebo. After eight weeks, each of the three active treatments was found to be better than placebo. The combined treatment was better than either CBT or medication alone, and those receiving CBT were also better able to sustain their improvements at follow-up when compared to those on medication alone. Furthermore, CBT, with or without medication, was felt by subjects, caregivers, and their doctors to be better than medication alone. Not surprisingly, subjects were also more satisfied with the cognitive-behavioral treatment approach.

Prescription medications used to treat insomnia include sleep-promoting substances, anti-anxiety medications, and sedating antidepressants.

Any medication that induces sleep can be considered a hypnotic drug, no matter what other actions it may have. However, some medications have received specific FDA approval to be marketed for the treatment of insomnia. By convention, these are known as "hypnotic" drugs, although in many cases they have other actions, such as the relief of anxiety. Equally, some drugs, such as antidepressants and anxiety-reducing agents, may be used for their sleep-enhancing effects. Table 17 lists examples of prescription medications with sleep-promoting effects.

Surgery and device-assisted treatments are much rarer. An example is a device that applies continuous positive airway pressure; called a CPAP machine, it can be very helpful for many people with sleep apnea.

Self-Help Treatments

Self-help treatments include over-the-counter sleep aids, herbal remedies, and good sleep hygiene. Whether you choose to pursue valerian or some other treatment, we strongly recommend that you look first to the habits that promote good sleep.

Review Your Sleep Hygiene First

For many of us just a few simple modifications to habits or to sleep environment can make a world of difference. *Sleep hygiene* is what we call the basic rules for promoting an environment conducive to sleep (see Table 18).

Table 17. Examples of Medications Often Prescribed to Promote Sleep

Class	Date developed	Drug (generic name)	Pros	Cons
Benzodiazepines	1950s, 1960s	Valium (diazepam) Librium (chlordiazepoxide) Restoril (temazepam) Dalmane (furazepam) Tranxene (clorazepate) Halcion (triazolam)	Rapid onset; effective; generally well tolerated	Risk of tolerance, dependence, and withdrawal; interactions with alcohol and other sedative drugs; can cause sexual dysfunction
Non-benzodiazepines	1990s	Ambien (zolpidem) Sonata (zaleplon)	Rapid onset; well-tolerated	More expensive
Sedating antidepressants	1950s, 1960s	Desyrel (trazodone) Sinequan (doxepin) Elavil (amitriptyline) Surmontil (trimipramine)	High level of efficacy	Multiple side effects; potential for drug interactions; dangerous in overdose
Sedating antihistamines	1960s	Atarax, Vistaril (hydroxyzine)	High level of efficacy	Side effects

What may appear to be a minor adjustment can frequently result in a major improvement. Sue found that skipping her afternoon nap and cutting out caffeine after noon returned her sleep pattern to normal after little more than a week. Bennett reevaluated his daily activities and noted that he was slow to start the day but picked up speed over time. As a result, he did his exercise routine and ate his largest meal toward the end of the day. So when he should be unwinding he was really just getting geared up to go. By forcing himself to exercise in the morning and by eating (and drinking) earlier and in moderation, he normalized his sleep patterns in a matter of weeks. Janet had been having sleep trouble for months, getting worse as job demands mounted. She found that with a trial of valerian in conjunction with self-discipline in avoiding snacks after dinner, recommitting herself to her yoga exercises, and reading quietly in the living room before retiring, she was feeling better in a week, with significant improvement overall in a few short weeks.

Over-the-Counter Medicines, or "Sleeping Pills"

Most people who just can't get the night's sleep they need turn first to over-the-counter sleep aids. These medicines are generally either products mar-

Table 18. Sleep Hygiene: Dos and Don'ts

Do
Maintain a regular sleep–wake schedule.
Keep up a steady program of daily exercise.
Insulate the bedroom from excessive light, noise, heat, cold.
If hungry, eat a light snack before retiring to bed.
Set aside time before turning in to work through emotion-laden concerns.

Don't
Engage in strenuous exercise immediately before bedtime.
Eat large meals before bedtime.
Consume alcohol, tobacco, or caffeinated drinks in the evening—or earlier in the day if you are particularly sensitive to these effects.
Eat other foods or use other products in the evening that contain tyramine (a substance that increases the release of a natural stimulant in our bodies), such as cheese and sauerkraut.
Take daytime naps.
Watch television in bed.
Frequently take a sleep aid, either bought over the counter or by prescription.
Use the bed as a stage to act out or work through emotional or sexual conflicts.

keted specifically for insomnia (e.g., Nytol, Sominex) or medicines recommended for other uses that have sleep-promoting side effects (e.g., many cold and allergy medicines). The active ingredients in most of these preparations are an anticholinergic (e.g., scopolamine), an antihistamine, and/or a salicylate. While these products may be used widely because of their accessibility, there is little hard scientific evidence to suggest that they are more effective than a placebo. In addition, these products are frequently associated with bothersome side effects, like dry mouth, daytime sedation, and other hangoverlike effects; more rarely, paradoxical excitement and confusion have been reported.

Valerian for Sleep

If you suffer from insomnia only occasionally—say, due to heightened job stress now and then—valerian may be an attractive choice for you. It allows you to treat yourself at a comparatively low cost. Most people tolerate it easily, suffering few side effects when they take it as directed. Valerian may also help you turn the corner if ongoing stress leaves you trapped in a pattern of increasing sleeplessness. *But you must resolve to use it on a temporary basis and to pursue nonmedicinal avenues to getting the rest you need.*

Colleen is typical of patients of ours who have found valerian an effective sleep aid. Colleen is a classic "supermom." Confident and capable, she somehow manages to chauffeur her three children to their many activities, care for her aging parents, hold her own household together, work part-time, and keep a 15-year marriage alive. Recently her husband embarked on a major career change, which will ultimately be best for the whole family but right now is placing additional responsibility on Colleen to supplement the family's income. Meanwhile, Colleen finds her brothers and sisters looking to her for strength in dealing with their eldest sister's fight against breast cancer and their middle brother's struggle with long-term depression.

Not too surprisingly, Colleen is finding the juggling act harder and harder to maintain. The stress and strain have taken their toll, most notably on her sleep. It usually takes her one to two hours to fall asleep, and she often wakes up once or twice in the middle of the night too. Worst of all, she feels wiped out in the morning, just when it is time to start the routine again.

A few years ago Colleen started taking an over-the-counter medicine to help her sleep. While it did help her fall asleep, she continued to wake up intermittently, and the medicine left her feeling groggy and "fuzzy-headed" in the morning, not quite herself until several hours and several cups of coffee into her day. And if she forgot to take it along with her when traveling or if she ran out, her sleep problems seemed even worse.

Colleen learned about valerian from a friend whose grandmother had grown up with valerian in Germany, where it had been a part of her family's medicine chest, next to the aspirin and laxatives. Colleen decided to give valerian a try. After one week she was falling asleep with greater ease, sleeping through the night, and awakening feeling refreshed and ready to attack the day—no more "medicine head"!

Anxious to avoid the dependence she had developed on the over-the-counter medicine, Colleen also took steps to educate herself about good sleep habits. She stopped staying up until the early morning hours doing laundry and instead enlisted the children's help on weekends. She became more aware of what and how much she was eating for dinner and cut out her evening cup of coffee in favor of a flavorful mug of herbal tea. She also took up yoga, which not only provided an opportunity for exercise and reflection but also gave her a little time all to herself. After taking valerian every night before bed for two to three weeks, Colleen found that her lifestyle changes were enough to help her sleep well on all but rare occasions. At times when she finds herself too wound up to fall asleep or to sleep through the night, she takes valerian for a day or so again. In general, though, she feels that now she has more control over her sleep at night, and consequently over her state of health and mind during the day.

Tony's stress did not build up gradually like Colleen's. It hit him over the head like a sledgehammer when, 10 months ago, Tony's father died after a massive heart attack that nobody saw coming. For the next few months Tony had increasing trouble sleeping. He would feel restless throughout the night, and it seemed that just when he fell asleep, it was time to get up again. He also tired more easily, dragging himself through the days, and noted trouble making decisions, finding that his thoughts would wander at times, often to memories of experiences he had had with his father. Tony's wife pleaded with him to see their family doctor. After a thorough evaluation, the doctor found Tony to be in good physical health although overtired.

After assuring Tony that he was experiencing the normal symptoms of grief, the doctor suggested that improved sleep would give Tony more energy and help him think clearly again. Though he would still feel sorrow for his father's death, he might find that he could get involved in and enjoy life again. Knowing that valerian was relatively benign, the doctor recommended it. For the first few weeks, Tony used the valerian nightly, gradually noting improvement in his sleep, energy, and concentration. His doctor advised him not to take valerian every night for more than six weeks, so now he has been using valerian only once a month or so, noting some sleep difficulty around Father's Day and just before his father's recent 60th birthday. His interest in carpentry, a hobby he had shared with his father, has been rekindled, and he has recently undertaken a project to turn their unfinished basement into a family room.

Harris considers sleeplessness a somewhat predictable, if unwelcome, part of his life at least once a year, when he has to make his presentation in front of the board of directors at the annual stockholders' meeting. As product design manager for a competitive software company that is a major player in the international market, Harris knows that he can be replaced by the next genius to come down the line at any time. Usually he is confident in his own proven abilities, but during the weeks leading up to the presentation he finds that as the pressure mounts his nightly hours of restful sleep decrease, robbing him of creativity and concentration when he can least afford the loss. Like Colleen, Harris has found that over-the-counter "sleeping pills" make him groggy, so after one or two days of insomnia he takes valerian two hours before bedtime. He cuts out his usual evening cocktail, and he's extra-diligent about working out every morning before heading for the office. He knows what being too wound up to sleep feels like to him, so once he's able to relax after work again—usually not until the stockholders' meeting has come and gone—he stops taking valerian but tries to keep up with his other sleep-promoting habits.

At this time we don't have much information on valerian's effectiveness in specific sleep disorders. As the preceding examples illustrate, valerian helps most with insomnia related to stress and anxiety.

How Do We Know Valerian Promotes Sleep?

Valerian's pharmacological history is typical of the circle that many medicinal herbs have traveled during the 20th century. A hundred years ago it was still common practice in much of the world to follow the tenets of folk medicine and take advantage of the medicinal properties of plants. However, things changed dramatically over the course of this century. In some cases it was the dwindling supplies of herbs, while in others it was the success of synthetic drugs and the benefits of patent protection that pushed interest in herbal remedies to the periphery. When the synthetic medicines proved to come with troublesome side effects and other baggage, interest in herbal medicines was revived.

In the case of valerian, supplies were exhausted around the time of World War II, when the herb was used to treat shell shock and other nervous conditions. Valerian continued in use until the consequent search for a manufactured alternative brought us the benzodiazepines in the late 1950s and 1960s, which were hailed for their effectiveness in treating insomnia and anxiety. But when the benzodiazepines were discovered to cause dependence, research efforts turned back to valerian.

Investigations undertaken in Europe, particularly in Germany, offered scientific evidence that valerian was a kinder, gentler alternative to the benzodiazepines. In place of the drowsiness, unsteadiness, sexual difficulties, and other impairments, along with addictive properties and drug and alcohol interactions, that accompanied the benzodiazepines, valerian seemed to produce almost no side effects and to lack addictive properties.

Valium and Valerian: No Relation

Because of the slight similarity in their names, many people have assumed that the prescription sedative Valium and the herb valerian are related. In fact, these products are very different, with unrelated chemical structures, although there is some evidence to suggest that valerian and Valium—perhaps the best known of the benzodiazepines—may share a chemical mechanism mediated by the brain chemical gamma-aminobutyric acid (GABA). So they are completely different, but they may have some of the same workings—which may explain why they are both effective in treating insomnia and mild anxiety.

Over the last several decades, evidence supporting the use of valerian has come from animal studies performed *in vitro* (in an artificial medium) and *in vivo* (in a living animal) and from human clinical studies. This research has included studies examining the individual constituents of valerian, as well as whole extracts of the herb, with very limited information on combined valerian products.

Animal Studies

Animal studies have revealed that valerian has a number of different effects, including sedative effects, modulation of neurochemical responses to stress and anxiety, anticonvulsant effects, muscle relaxation, and antidepressant effects. But the research has fallen far short of telling us everything we need to know. Different parts of the herb, from the essential oil, to various chemicals such as valerenic acid, to the whole valerian extract, taken from the root stock, have been found to have medicinal qualities. We clearly have a lot more to learn about where the herb's various medicinal powers come from and how the chemicals in the plant work together. More details on how valerian works—as far as we know today—are provided on page 215.

Nor do we know exactly where valerian exerts its powers in the human body. In animal studies the herb has demonstrated neurochemical effects in the central nervous system, as well as muscle-relaxing properties that seem to work directly on the muscle tissue and not through the nervous system. Also, different studies have examined different *Valeriana* species. Finally, many of these animal studies were performed *in vitro* (in an artificial medium), and it is unclear if these effects would also be observed *in vivo* (in a living animal).

Clinical Studies

Human research has focused on the sleep-promoting and potential calmative effects, as well as the possible performance-impairing actions, of valerian. These studies have included healthy volunteers, those suffering from insomnia, and those suffering from anxiety-stress reactions. A variety of formulations and preparations have been studied, such as single valerian preparations and preparations combining valerian extracts with other herbs.

Ten controlled studies of valerian have been published. Three of these studies were conducted in healthy people (Balderer and Borbely, 1985; Leathwood and Chauffard, 1983, 1984), and seven in patients with sleep disturbances (Donath et al., 1996; Jansen, 1977; Kamm-Kohl et al., 1984; Lindahl and Lindwall, 1989; Schulz et al., 1994; Schulz and Jobert, 1995; Vorbach et al., 1996). Four studies used the same aqueous extract; the other six used various dried, ethanol, or syrup extracts. Dosages ranged from 270 mg to 1,215 mg, and treatment lasted from one day to 30 days. In the brief trials lasting from one to four days, healthy subjects were assessed after receiving valerian, a comparator medication(s), or placebo; in the one four-day crossover study, each subject received two doses of valerian and of placebo, taking one dose per day.

Effects of Valerian on Sleep. Among healthy subjects, those receiving valerian tended to fall asleep more quickly compared to those receiving placebo, with a significant reduction in time taken to fall asleep (called *sleep latency*) observed in subjects taking valerian and with substantially improved sleep quality. Valerian was generally quite well tolerated.

Findings from these studies demonstrate that after one dose of the herb and compared to a placebo or an active comparator, valerian can improve sleep onset and sleep quality in healthy people. While these findings are interesting, they say nothing about the effectiveness of valerian treatment over several days and weeks in individuals with sleep problems—whether it works or not and, if so, in what ways.

Findings from the longer controlled studies shed some light on these issues. These larger controlled studies were conducted in adults of all ages, all with some form of sleep difficulty. In each investigation, the efficacy of valerian was evaluated using standard subjective (self-rated) and objective (interviewer- or physician-rated) rating scales. Kamm-Kohl and colleagues (1984) conducted a study of 80 elderly hospitalized patients with behavior disorders of nervous origin, which included difficulties falling asleep and sleeping through the night and easy fatigability due to impaired sleep. Subjects were treated daily with 270 mg of valerian or placebo over two weeks. Significant improvements were reported in sleep, as well as in mood and behavior. The medication was well tolerated.

In a more recent study, Vorbach et al. (1996) studied 121 adults with sleep disturbances of at least four weeks' duration. Participants were treated with 600 mg of either valerian or placebo for four weeks. No improvement was noted initially; however, after two weeks of treatment, significant global improvement was observed in the valerian group, but without meaningful changes in the other measures. After four weeks, significant improvement was noted on all measures of sleep and mood in favor of valerian. These findings are particularly noteworthy because they suggest that the sleep-promoting effects of valerian are different from those of the prescription sedatives and hypnotics. Specifically, full therapeutic benefit from valerian is probably not attained in less than two to four weeks of treatment. Consumers need to keep this in mind when using valerian and continue to give the herb a full two- to four-week trial before calling it quits if it does not seem to work. However, valerian can also work quite quickly, even after a single dose. As yet, we can't explain these different types of activity.

Effects of Valerian on Performance and Alertness. For some people, a major downfall of many prescription sedatives and over-the-counter medicines is that they can cloud your thinking, making you feel less "sharp," and may also slow your reaction time. Valerian may well be a good alternative, and has been compared to other calmative herbs and to prescription sedatives concerning these effects. In one study, researchers concerned about risk of accident proneness when using valerian set out to assess the herb's acute sedative effects and impact on vigilance (Gerhard et al., 1991). A commercial valerian preparation, Valverde, containing valerian, lemon balm, passionflower, and pestilence wort, was compared to 3 mg of bromazepine (a benzodiazepine) and placebo in 60 healthy male participants. No difference was found for either active treatment compared to placebo or in side effects reported. In a subsequent study, this group examined the effect of two plant-based sedatives on vigilance, with particular application to recommendations concerning potential hazards in driving or operating heavy machinery (Gerhard et al., 1996). Eighty healthy subjects were treated with either a valerian syrup, tablets containing valerian and hops, flunitrazepam (a standard benzodiazepine hypnotic used in Europe), or placebo. Assessments included self-ratings of well-being and objective ratings of cognitive and psychomotor performance, as well as evaluation of tolerance. On the morning following treatment, impaired performance was observed in the flunitazepam group only on both subjective and objective ratings, whereas those receiving a valerian formulation noted feeling better, more alert, and active. Valerian was quite well tolerated, with only 10 percent of those receiving valerian extract or a combination product containing hops noting adverse effects. This rate was equal to that reported by the placebo group and far less than those in the benzodiazepine comparator group, 50 percent of whom reported adverse effects. In a few cases, there was slight impairment of vigilance one to two hours after taking valerian syrup extract. With the dried valerian and hops extract, there was some slowed processing of complex information, but performance wasn't impaired the following morning. Based on their findings, the authors concluded that hangover effects need not be a concern, although noting that a slight reduction in performance may be observed in the first few hours following ingestion.

Effects of Valerian on Stress. In recent years several other studies have looked at valerian in the treatment of stress conditions. In a double-blind crossover study, a mixture of valerian and hops was evaluated in reducing stress that develops in traffic (Moser, 1981). Significant improvement was noted in drivers' reports of stress experienced and in objective measures of reaction time. Another double-blind study looked at the effect of valerian on physiological activation (as measured by pulse changes), performance (solving math problems in front of a group, as well as written calculations), and mood (Kohnen and Oswald, 1988). Forty-eight healthy volunteers received either 100 mg of valerian extract, 20 mg of propranolol (a beta-adrenergic agent), or a combination of the two. In contrast to propranolol, valerian was not associated with reductions in physiological arousal under stress (heart rate actually increased), but it did show improvement in anxiety and mood. No sedative effects were observed with valerian, as might be expected at such a small dose. A third controlled study (Bourin et al., 1997) has looked at the effects of a combination product called Euphytose (containing extracts of *Cretaegus, Ballota, Passiflora, Valeriana, Cola,* and *Paullinia*) in treating 182 people with adjustment disorders with anxious mood. Euphytose was significantly better than placebo for anxiety. It is unclear, however, exactly what constituents were responsible for the observed improvement.

How convincing is the research evidence we have today? A mounting body of data supports the calmative effects of whole valerian extracts, but these studies had their limitations. Were depression and other potential causes of sleep difficulty ruled out? Were subjects taking other medications or using alcohol before or during the study? (This would impact the effectiveness of the study treatments.) Was the control treatment selected an appropriate one? Was the herb standardized, and were adequate doses used? Were the patients and objective assessors truly blinded to the treatment administered? Such questions notwithstanding, these studies all provide encouraging evidence as to the value of valerian in the relief of insomnia, with some further suggestion of an anti-anxiety and stress-modulating effect.

Relative to other herbals, valerian may perhaps be viewed as the herb of first choice for treating insomnia, since it is by far the best studied in this regard. In comparison to standard hypnotic drugs, it is perhaps less powerful but at the same time enjoys the advantage of fewer side effects and perhaps less impairment in performance and vigilance.

My health food store is loaded with natural sleep aids. Is valerian better than all the others?

Over the years a number of other herbs have been claimed to possess hypnotic properties. The most popular ones include lemon balm (*Melissa officinalis*), passionflower (*Passiflora incarnata*), kava kava (*Piper methysticum;* see Chapter 2), hops (*Humulus lupulus*), St. John's wort (*Hypericum perforatum;* see Chapter 1), and chamomile (*Chamaemelum nobile*). Another natural product that has been shown to be helpful in some people with sleep disturbances is melatonin. Unfortunately, at this time we do not really know how valerian compares with any of these.

If valerian is good, is valerian plus one of the other sleep-promoting herbs even better?

A number of herbal mixtures have been recommended over the centuries to treat insomnia. In fact, up until 1990, the majority of herbs used in Germany were sold in combination. Products containing valerian in combination with other sedating herbs are becoming increasingly popular among U.S. consumers. Herbs commonly combined with *Valeriana officinials* include hops, passionflower, lemon balm, and kava. While the evidence is only anecdotal, some people believe that the combination of valerian with lemon balm produces a more rapid hypnotic effect than valerian alone. The German Commission E has assessed a number of combination products and has given approval for several fixed combinations (see Table 19).

Would valerian be a good choice for my 70-year-old aunt, who rarely sleeps through the night? She is otherwise a healthy woman.

Sleep length varies naturally with age. In infancy, we sleep deeply for up to two-thirds of each 24-hour period. Following adolescence, while sleep occupies only a third of our time, it continues to be deep and fulfilling. Over the years, in the fifth and sixth decades and thereafter, our sleep becomes increasingly shallower and of shorter duration. Data from several studies of healthy elderly people with sleep trouble suggests that valerian can be effective and safe. However, it is important to remember that older individuals metabolize medications differently and are frequently more sensitive to side effects, so your aunt should start with a lower dose than you would use.

Table 19. Fixed Combinations of Valerian Root Approved
by the German Commission E

Fixed combination of drug	Uses	Dosage
Passionflower, Valerian root, lemon balm	Conditions of unrest, difficulty in falling asleep due to nervousness	Individual components must each be present at 30 to 50% of the daily dosage given in the monographs for the individual herbs.
Valerian root and hops	Nervous sleeping disorders, conditions of unrest	Individual components must be at a concentration of 50 to 75% of the dosage given in the monograph for the single herbs.
Valerian root, hops, lemon balm	Difficulty in falling asleep due to nervousness, unrest	In a combination of two of these components, the individual components must be present at 50 to 75% of the daily dosage recommended in the monographs for the individual herbs. In combinations of all three components, each component must be at 30 to 50% of the daily dosage recommended in the monographs for the single herbs.
Valerian root, hops, passionflower	Difficulty in falling asleep due to nervousness, unrest	In a combination of two of these components, the individual components must be present at 50 to 75% of the daily dosage recommended in the monographs for the individual herbs. In combinations of all three components, each component must be at 30 to 50% of the daily dosage recommended in the monographs for the single herbs.

Note. Information from German Commission E Monographs (1998).

My 10-year-old daughter is high-strung, nervous, and temperamental. If we try to get her to go to bed at a time when she'll get enough sleep before getting up for school, she ends up lying in bed staring at the ceiling or fidgeting until 11:00 P.M. anyway. Could an herbal remedy like valerian relax her enough to fall asleep without harming her in any way?

The information we have on the use of valerian in children is largely limited to experiences of individual practitioners and consumers. Only one published uncontrolled study of valerian in sleep disturbance has included children. Two European countries have approved its use in children—for the treatment of sleep disorders in Belgium and for nervous or minor sleep disorders in France. Authorities in the United States, however, believe that there is insufficient data to determine its safety and efficacy in children and have therefore not approved its use for those under 18 years of age at this time. We would not recommend it for children until more information about its efficacy and safety is available.

I think valerian is terrific and have been recommending it to all my friends—at least until one friend who is pregnant said she couldn't take anything at all until the baby was born, despite the fact that she's exhausted from lack of sleep. Who should I not recommend it to?

As with other herbs and medications, particular caution should be exercised by several groups. Certainly anyone who is pregnant, suspects she might be pregnant, or is breastfeeding should talk to her doctor before taking valerian or any other herb. People with chronic medical conditions, particularly those with conditions requiring regular use of prescription medication and medical follow-up, should consult their physician before using valerian or any other dietary supplement. The same recommendation applies to the elderly, given the concerns cited earlier.

An herbalist I know suggested that valerian might relieve symptoms of depression that I've been feeling. Should I try it?

We have a lot more evidence suggesting that St. John's wort would be the herb of choice for treating depression, but valerian might very well help too. There is some preliminary scientific evidence to suggest that some *Valeriana* species may possess antidepressant properties. Two controlled human studies (Kamm-Kohl et al., 1984; Vorbach et al., 1996)in geriatric subjects with sleep disturbances have also provided evidence to suggest that *Valeriana officinalis* may have antidepressant effects. In the more recent of these two studies, participants reported significant improvements in mood and well-being after only two weeks of treatment, whereas the full sleep-promoting effects were not experienced until the end of four weeks of treatment. Together, the findings from these studies suggest that valerian may also have intrinsic antidepressant effects. This is an area that warrants further investigation, but we know of no studies being done at this time. In the meantime, however, clinicians in Germany may recommend taking valerian along with St. John's wort, noting safety from their local experience, should you wish to try that approach.

I'm being treated for recurrent urinary tract infections (UTI), which my doctors says are probably responsible for my insomnia, and I have a friend who's having trouble sleeping because of her chronic pain. Could valerian help either of us sleep?

The German Commission E monographs, the best compilation of data we have so far, report no drug interactions associated with valerian and no contraindications for its use. This means it should be safe for those who have medical conditions like your UTI and your friend's chronic pain. But that doesn't mean it will work. Studies to date have investigated the effects of valerian in healthy adults and in those with sleep disturbances. No published studies have systematically investigated valerian in treating sleep difficulties in people with primary psychological or medical problems.

As we noted earlier, if you are under a doctor's care for a chronic medical or emotional condition, whether or not you are taking a prescription medication, you should consult your physician before self-medicating with valerian. What we know about herb–drug interactions comes from relatively small and homogeneous clinical populations, as described earlier. As the use of valerian grows, the responses of larger and more heterogeneous populations—the young and the old, the healthy and the sick—will tell us more about potential toxicities from herb–herb and herb–drug interactions. Also, disrupted sleep may be a sign of a change in your condition or a side effect of a medication. Your physician should know about your insomnia in case an adjustment or change in medication is in order.

Valerian really helped me get back into a healthy sleeping pattern, and I haven't taken it for a few weeks. But I'm worried that my insomnia will come back, because I can't afford to lose sleep like that again. Would it be a good idea to keep taking valerian, maybe at a lower dose, to make sure I keep sleeping well?

To date no evidence suggests that valerian has preventive or protective effects, and we wouldn't recommend taking it for any continuous period beyond six weeks, even if you are still suffering from insomnia. Preparations containing very large quantities of valepotriates, one of the active constituents of valerian, may actually have harmful effects. This issue is discussed further in the section "Toxicity and Overdose" (see page 220).

To be on the safe side, when shopping for valerian, look for products that contain *Valeriana officinalis*. This should not be too difficult since products with *Valeriana officinalis* predominate in the American herbal market. We agree with the established recommendation against long-term use of valerian, that is, beyond six weeks. A limited period of use is recommended in part because the studies performed to date have been of relatively brief duration and we know that valerian is safe to use under these conditions. In addition, as with other sleep aids, chronic, long-term use without medical supervision is discouraged because of the concerns for developing psychological dependence on the treatment and for potentially masking another treatable cause of the sleep disturbance.

Can valerian help treat the effects of jet lag?

So far the published literature contains nothing about the use of valerian for treating jet lag, and it seems unlikely that the herb would help. Jet leg results from a disruption in the 24-hour sleep–wake cycle that reconciles itself within several days after you've returned to your usual time zone. Because longer controlled studies showed that the full benefits of valerian did not appear until after four weeks of treatment, it is unlikely that valerian has the kind of action that would speed up the adjustment process.

❧ HOW VALERIAN WORKS

Valerian is native to Europe and temperate zones of Asia but is now cultivated all around the Northern Hemisphere, from Europe to North America, from Russia to Japan. Commercially traded species include *Valeriana wallichii* (syn. *Valeriana jatamansii*), *Valeriana fauriei*, and *Valeriana edulis*, though *Valeriana officinalis* is used in most preparations you'll find on retail shelves in the United States. As we'll discuss on page 225, it's very important that the product you purchase be standardized to provide a certain amount of the active sedative, because the chemical composition of the plants varies tremendously, from one species to the next and from one plant to another. The product you buy can even vary depending on what part of the plant has been used to make it, though the vast majority of preparations are made from the root stock, where the sedating properties of the plant are believed to lie.

Determining how and why valerian's chemical makeup varies is only one vexing task facing scientists today. More important is finding out exactly how valerian works. If we can figure out which of the herb's constituents are responsible for valerian's sleep-promoting properties and by which mechanisms they operate, we may be able to synthesize valerian's powers in the same way that scientists who isolated acetylsalicylic acid from willow bark gave us the "wonder drug" we call *aspirin*. Unfortunately, centuries after being added to the world's pharmacopeia, valerian remains an enigma. In biblical times valerian's medicinal properties were believed to be related to its bitter and aromatic properties. This theory persisted at least until World War II, when the fact that valerian's "action has been attributed to its unpleasant smell" led one observer to speculate that "deodorised preparations cannot possess any activity due to their valerian content" (Martindale, 1941).

Since the beginning of the 20th century, numerous observations and studies have considered the sedative qualities of both whole valerian extract and specific constituents (listed in Table 20) in an effort to pin down the workings of the herb, but the results have always been inconsistent. In the early 1900s scientists had yet to isolate specific chemical constituents of the herb, but generally they believed that valerian's power to sedate lay in the essential oil, which exists almost exclusively in the rootstock. Once components of the essential oil had been isolated, animal studies of its more than 150 compounds began. Of particular interest was valerenic acid, a definitive chemical component of *Valeriana officinalis*, according to the *European Pharmacopeia* (1985). Valerenic acid has demonstrated substantial sedative and antispasmodic activity, but it apparently produces only about one-third of the sedative effects of parent valerian.

To find out what ingredient(s) was(were) responsible for the balance of sedative effects, scientists turned their attention to other constituents, particularly the valepotriate iridoids. Again the findings were inconclusive. Calmative effects were found in some animal studies but not in others. Nevertheless, belief that valepotriates are the source of valerian's sedative properties remains strong. One brand of valerian used widely in Germany as a mild to moderate sedative is marketed under the name Valmane; it contains a standardized extract of didrovaltrate (80 percent), valtrate (15 percent), and acevaltrate (5 percent) (Houghton, 1997), three of the four

Table 20. Chemical Constituents of *Valeriana Officinalis*

1. Essential oil (0.2–1.0%)[a]
   - Monterpenes
     (–)–Bornyl isovalerenate
     (–)–Bornyl isovalerneic acid
   - Sesquiterpenes
     Valerenic acid (0.1–0.9%)
     2-Hydroxyvalerenic acid
     2-Acetoxyvalerenic acid

2. Iridoids
   - Valepotriates (0.2–2.0%)
     Isovaltrate (≤ 46%)
     Valtrate (80–90%[b])
     Isovaleroxyhydroxydidrovaltrate (10–20%)
     Acevaltrate
     Didrovaltrate

3. Alkaloids
   - Actinidine
   - Valerianine
   - Alpha-methylpyrrylketone

4. Caffeic acid derivatives
   - Chologenic acid

Note. Except for valtrate, data from *Herbal PDR* (1998).
[a]Contains over 150 compounds.
[b]Data from Samuelsson (1992) and Stahl and Schild (1971).

principal valepotriates in *Valeriana officinalis*. Despite such confidence, we still don't understand which valepotriate (and its derivatives), if any, contributes to the sedative activity we associate with valerian.

The alkaloids listed as the third major component actually exist in only very small amounts in valerian and are not believed to contribute appreciably to its sedative properties. Several amino acids have also been found in *Valeriana officinalis*, as have phenylpropanoids and fatty acids, including linoleic acid, an unsaturated fatty acid found in our daily diets. These constituents remain under investigation as the search for the biologically active components of valerian continues.

What we are left with, then, is a growing sense that multiple components probably contribute to valerian's biological activity and that, as with many other herbal remedies, the whole may be greater than the sum of its parts. Thanks to a natural synergism that may take place within the plant, we may never be able to reduce valerian to a synthetic sleep aid on the order of aspirin. This could be both good news and bad: we may be receiving unknown benefits from some unidentified ingredient or mechanism when we take a remedy based on whole valerian extract, but if we choose valerian as our sleep aid, we may also have to live with the vagaries of varying potency and efficacy that come with living plants, an issue that may be made more acceptable, however, with the development of regulatory standardization.

As to how valerian exerts its anti-anxiety effects, we are even more in the dark. Does valerian reduce anxiety as a primary effect of the herb or simply as a secondary effect of getting good, sound sleep? We really don't know, and this remains an issue to be investigated further, but at this time we are unaware of any specific ongoing research in this area.

Side Effects and Other Risks

Side Effects

As we noted earlier, the effectiveness of prescription sleep aids sometimes comes at a cost that not everyone is willing to, or should, take. There may be potential for abuse and dependence; they may cause side effects that can interfere with your ability to think clearly and perform physically; their interactions with alcohol and other medications can be serious if not used as directed. A number of sleeping medicines are considered controlled substances by the Drug Enforcement Agency and are available by prescription only. Even over-the-counter sleeping pills often leave the user feeling hungover or groggy the next day.

Valerian has fewer side effects than both prescription sedatives and over-the-counter sleep aids. Acute side effects are rarely reported with valerian-only products but may include mild headaches, nausea, nervousness, and palpitations. It is important to note, however, that controlled studies to date are rather vague about the rate of side effects, reporting only that they are "low." For valerian and other herbs we have nothing as precise as the numerical data we have for adverse effects of pharmaceutical agents.

After taking valerian and getting a good night's sleep, most people report feeling rested and refreshed in the morning, but a very small minority of consumers has reported feeling groggy or a bit slowed upon awakening. If you tend to be very sensitive to medication side effects, you may want to start at a lower dose, such as 150 mg before bedtime, and see how you feel the following morning. Also beware of using valerian inappropriately, because adverse effects such as morning sleepiness are likely to be increased if you take valerian in doses higher than those recommended or in combination with alcohol, prescription sedatives, or other sleep medication.

Multiherb preparations may carry greater potential risk for adverse events. In one case series, four patients taking proprietary products containing multiple ingredients, including valerian and skullcap, developed liver changes indicative of toxicity (MacGregor et al., 1989). The fact that these liver abnormalities resolved over time after discontinuation of the herbal products suggests that those products may in fact have caused the abnormalities. However, it remains unknown whether this was related to the valerian, the skullcap, the combination, or some other factor.

Effects of Long-Term Use

In general, the regular use of any sleep aid—prescription, over-the-counter, or herbal—is ill-advised, for a number of reasons. For example, persistently disrupted sleep may be a sign of another underlying problem that needs to be addressed. In addition, taking sleep aids regularly for a long time can lead to psychological dependence, and, in the case of prescription sedatives and hypnotics, such as the benzodiazepines, physiological dependence or even addiction. While psychological dependence is not a true addiction, feeling that you are unable to sleep without a medicinal aid can be very uncomfortable and make it even more difficult to sleep without some type of hypnotic agent.

Concerning valerian in particular, according to observations made over the years, longtime, chronic users of large doses may experience symptoms such as headache, excitability and mental agitation, restlessness, nausea and diarrhea, palpitations, and slowed reaction time with dulling of senses. It is said that Adolf Hitler was a valerian addict and regularly took large and excessive doses.

To date, however, no reports of valerian causing physical or psychological dependence have been published. The only published report (Garges et al., 1998) we have so far that even suggests the potential for dependence following long-term use of valerian involved a man who had taken valerian for many years on a daily basis at very high doses to help him "relax and sleep." When he was admitted to the hospital for a surgical procedure and his valerian was discontinued, he developed a clinical picture suggestive of benzodiazepine withdrawal. It is important to point out in this case, however, that this patient had a number of significant medical problems requiring treatment with many medications. Therefore, this single case is not enough evidence to show that valerian caused withdrawal symptoms, but it strengthens our recommendations to use valerian only on an intermittent and short-term basis and at recommended doses in treating insomnia and to check with your physician if you have a condition requiring regular medical follow-up or medication.

Toxicity and Overdose

In general, valerian is believed to be quite safe when taken according to the recommended guidelines. The German Commission E monograph on valerian reports that there are no side effects, contraindications, or known drug interactions with *Valeriana officinalis*. Still, it's wise to keep in mind that every substance has the potential for toxicity. Paracelsus (1493–1541) recognized this danger when he observed 500 years ago that the only difference between a medicine and a poison is the dose. A general guideline when taking any medication that can cause drowsiness, such as valerian, is to use care in the daytime while driving, using heavy machinery, or when engaged in other activities with the potential for danger with sedation.

A small but growing body of evidence suggests that products containing very large concentrations of valepotriates and their decomposition products should be avoided. A group of Dutch scientists examined the potential of valerian and its constituents to cause cells to die (Bos et al., 1998). They found a clear relationship between the valepotriate contents of freshly prepared tinctures and their toxicity, whereby fresh tinctures of *Valeriana edulis* were found to be the most toxic, containing the highest levels of valepotriates. In contrast, *Valeriana officinalis* was the least toxic, with the greatest reduction in toxicity over time. The authors point out, however, that whether these findings would be borne out in humans remains unclear. Other reports from animal studies (Schulz et al., 1998; Tufik et al., 1994) suggest that products with Mexican and Indian valerian (containing high concentrations of valepotriates and their by-products) should be avoided due to concerns for potential cell damage found in rats.

The information available regarding overdose with valerian is limited. One case report (Willey et al., 1995) has been published, involving an 18-year-old girl who attempted suicide by ingesting 40 to 50 470-mg capsules of valerian (equivalent to 18.8 to 23.5 grams of the herb). Thirty minutes later she experienced fatigue, abdominal cramping, chest tightness, tremulousness of hands and feet, and lightheadedness. Three hours later, in the emergency room, her pupils were dilated and she had a fine hand tremor, but her blood tests were normal. Twenty-four hours later, after being given two doses of activated charcoal to promote removal of any residual valerian from her gastrointestinal tract, her symptoms had disappeared completely. Unfortunately, no further follow-up information was available to see how she did down the road. Findings from one small study (Chan, 1998), however, did not find evidence of residual toxic effects.

Valerian with Alcohol

Though alcohol has been known to have dangerous interactions with prescription sedatives such as the benzodiazepines, valerian does not seem to have the same type of interaction. Findings from one double-blind, placebo-controlled trial (Albrecht et al., 1995) assessing the effects of a commercial preparation containing dried extracts of *Valeriana* and *Melissa* (640 mg twice per day) on mental and physical performance when driving found that valerian did not worsen impairment due to alcohol at a blood level of 0.5 percent. In an animal study conducted 30 years ago (von Eikstedt, 1969), investigators examined the interactions between alcohol and either valepotriates or either of two benzodiazepines (Valium and Librium). Mice treated with the combination of valepotriates and alcohol actually demonstrated less impairment in one performance measure, along with prolonged anesthesia, whereas alcohol was more toxic in combination with either of the benzodiazepines. It is not clear, however, if these findings would be replicated in humans.

While specific interactions between valerian and alcohol have not been reported, remember that insomnia can be caused or worsened by alcohol consumption, and it is best to avoid alcohol altogether until your sleep problems subside.

Drug Interactions

It is important to remember that many substances have psychoactive properties (i.e., they affect the brain and behavior) and therefore should be taken with caution. Interaction between substances could either inactivate one or both or enhance or exaggerate their effects, possibly with the buildup of a substance to a toxic level in the body.

The literature pertaining to interactions between valerian and other drugs is scant but will likely expand in the future with the growing use of the herb and as standards for adverse event reporting are developed. In several animal studies (Bounthanh et al., 1980; Hendricks et al., 1985; Rosencrans et al., 1961), valerian has potentiated the effects of barbiturates, a class of medications with sedating and antiseizure properties. Atropine, a centrally acting anticholinergic medication, has been observed to reduce the blood-pressure-lowering effects of valerian (Rosencrans et al., 1961).

How quickly does valerian work?

Some people taking valerian for sleep trouble will note effects almost immediately. Others, however, may not experience the full sleep-promoting effects of valerian until after several weeks of treatment. Even if the full sedative benefit does not appear immediately, other positive effects, including improvement in mood and general well-being, can show up early in treatment.

❦ HOW TO USE VALERIAN

What Type of Preparation Is Best?

As with other herbs, valerian is available in a variety of forms, including capsules or pills containing dried powdered root, liquid extracts and tinctures, and infusions or teas. There is no "best" way to take valerian, so use a form that suits you best. Some people prefer the ease and convenience of a pill or capsule. At the end of a long day, others may opt to drink a beverage or a warm cup of tea in a quiet, relaxing environment. Some people who tend to wake up in the middle of the night and need something to help them fall back to sleep swear by tinctures, claiming that since they are the most potent they work fastest (a response that may be facilitated by a substantial alcohol content!).

You may notice as you shop that valerian is not available in time-release form. Remember that its primary use is for insomnia, in which case you would want it to take effect relatively quickly. Using a time-released preparation under these circumstances seems to be illogical though it could potentially have utility in treating anxiety and stress. In addition, time-release formulations are expensive and time-consuming to develop and, up to this point, have not been a focus of the infant herbal industry.

When to Take Valerian

At what time of day you take valerian will depend on why you are using it. For insomnia, it's best to take it 30 to 90 minutes before retiring. For mild anxiety that lasts throughout the day, you can split the day's total amount into two or three doses—perhaps one on the morning, one in the afternoon, and one at bedtime. Don't be confused by the fact that some labels will direct you to take one dose before bed and others will tell you to take a number of doses throughout the day. These instructions are obviously based on the manufacturer's assumptions about your reason for using the herb.

We have no evidence that it matters whether you take it with food or on an empty stomach.

Determining Dosages

Effective dose may vary from one person to the next; what is right for you may not be effective for your neighbor. In controlled trials of valerian in healthy subjects and in those with sleep disturbances, doses ranging from 300 mg to 900 mg were shown to be helpful in promoting sleep. Most practitioners recommend doses between 300 and 600 mg. If you are a first-time valerian user, it is a good idea to start at the lower end of the dosage range, taking the herb an hour or so before retiring. If the lower dose is ineffective, you then have room to increase the dose within the recommended range.

To treat mild anxiety states, many herbalists suggest taking valerian more than once a day. A smaller dose of, say, 100 to 300 mg may be taken in the morning and during the day, followed by an evening dose of 300 to 600 mg roughly an hour before going to bed.

Dosing has not been widely studied systematically and scientifically. Generally speaking, recommendations for dosing vary among practitioners and are based largely on the practitioners' experience with different preparations and for different health applications. A list of dosing instructions included in a number of available texts is summarized in Table 21 and may provide some guidance on how and when to take valerian.

Table 21. Summary of Dosage Recommendations for *Valeriana Officinalis*

Source	Dried root/rhizome	Extract	Tincture	Infusion or tea	Bath
Brown (1996)		*Stdzd*: ≥ 0.5% essential oil, 300–400 mg, one to two times a day. *For insomnia*: 300–500 mg, 1 hour before bedtime. *For mild anxiety*: 150–300 mg in morning and 300–500 mg before bedtime			
Murray (1995)	1–2 g, 30–45 min before bedtime	1:1 fluid extract, 1–2 ml. *Stdzd*: 0.8% valerenic acid, 150–300 mg, 30–45 min before bedtime	1:5—4–6 ml, 30–45 min before bedtime	1–2 mg, 30–45 min before bedtime	
Schulz et al. (1998)	2 g (approximately 400 mg) of 5:1 herb extract				
Upton et al. (1999)	2–3 g	1:1 flue extract—0.5–1.0 ml, one to three times a day	1:5—1–3 ml, one to four times a day	Cold or hot infusion: 1 cup or as needed	100 g
Newall et al. (1996)	0.3–1.0 g three times a day	0.3–1.0 ml	0.3–1.0 ml	0.3–1.0 g, three times a day	
Blumenthal et al. (1998)		Equivalent to 2–3 g taken one to several times a day	½–1 tsp (1–3 ml), one to several times a day	2–3 g/cup, taken one to several times a day	100 g
Herbal PDR (1998)		Equivalent to 2–3 g taken one to several times a day	1:5—15–20 drops in water, taken one to several times a day	1 cup, taken one to several times a day	

Are the dosing recommendations the same for older adults as for younger ones?

As a rule of thumb, healthy people over age 65 should start at lower doses (100 to 150 mg) and increase the dose slowly if it is ineffective. Use should be discontinued immediately at the first sign of any problems or discomforts and their primary care physician consulted.

Choosing a Brand

Which product to buy becomes a tougher and tougher question as store shelves fill with more and more choices. You need to consider the same criteria as for other herbs (see the Introduction), but in the case of valerian you need to take special care to determine potency and freshness. These issues, plus what we know about the valerian products available at this time, are discussed below.

Standardized Potency

One way to look at potency is as a measure of the strength of the product. This is determined by a number of factors including the dose (e.g., number of milligrams per unit dose), standardization, and age of the product. First, the dosage can vary widely from one brand to the next—in dose per pill (mg per pill) as well as in recommended daily dose (pills per day). Second, presumably, a brand standardized to a given percent of valerenic acid will be more potent than one without any standardization—or at least we have more confidence in the potency and consistency of the standardized brand. Third, products may lose some of their potency over time, and it is therefore important to examine expiration dates when buying herbal remedies and over-the-counter medications. While we have no real way to know of an herb's potency without sophisticated chemical analysis, we are at least guided by the expiration date listed on the product, which indicates a satisfactory degree of potency. Details of what to look for follow.

As we explained earlier, the contents of the essential oil, one of the pharmacologically active constituents, vary between valerian subspecies as well as within a given species from year to year due to differences in growing conditions, age of the root, harvesting times (generally between August and October for medicinal quality *Valeriana officinalis*), and drying techniques.

Unless the product you buy states—and lives up to the claim—that it has been standardized to a certain strength of active ingredients, be suspicious.

The average yield of essential oil is 0.4 to 0.6 percent, again, varying within and between species. For example, Japanese *Valeriana officinalis* var. *latifolia* has been recorded to contain from 0.5 to 6.0 percent essential oil, while *Nardostachys jatamansi* DC contains about 4 percent. The essential oil content of medicinal valerian (e.g., European *Valeriana officinalis)* ranges from 0.2 to 1.0 percent, with pharmacopoeial standards generally requiring 0.5 percent essential oil based on dry weight.

Carefully dried *Valeriana officinalis* also contains at least 0.8 percent valepotriates (Samuelsson, 1992), but rarely more than 1.2 percent. European *Valeriana officinalis* contains 0.4 to 0.6 percent valepotriates.

Most pharmacopoeial standards recommend that valerian extracts be standardized to at least 0.5 percent valerenic acid. We conducted a survey of herbal products available in a number of different retail stores (health food store, grocery store, large discount store), the results of which are shown in Table 22. Of the products we surveyed, only three were standardized at or above the 0.5 percent valerenic acid level—to 0.8 percent valerenic acid—1 to 0.2 percent, and 1 to 0.1 percent (note that these latter products were in combination with other sedating herbs). The other half of the products (five) were not standardized at all (or if they were, it was not listed on the label!).

In determining whether the product might be potent enough to help you, also check to see if there are other ingredients in the product. If the valerenic acid content is less than 0.5 percent, but the preparation contains other herbs with sleep-promoting properties, it may still be effective. Table 19 presented combinations approved by Germany's Commission E, based on the government standard that each medicinally active component in the preparation contributes to the product's effectiveness and safety. Unfortunately, however, at this time we do not have scientific study data to support the effectiveness of such combinations in treating sleep disturbances or anxiety.

Valerian products contain both valerenic acid and valepotriates. Initially the belief was that valerenic acid was the "active" component, so standardization was based on this component. Over time, exactly what is the active component has become less clear, but products are still standardized to valerenic acid. On some preparations you may also see standardization of valepotriates and essential oil content, but pharmacopeial standards use the valerenic acid content.

The components of *Valeriana officinalis* believed to possess its medici-

Table 22. Comparisons of Different Brands of Valerian Available in Three Different Retail Stores (November 1998)

Store	Brand	Dose/pill	Pills/day	Standardized	Other ingredients	Expiration date	Cost/day
1	A	400 mg	2–8 as needed	No	Yes (2)	Yes	$0.16–0.64
	B	530 mg	1–2 as needed	Yes (0.8%)	No	Yes	$0.11–0.22
2	C	400 mg	2–8 as needed	No	Yes (2)	Yes	$0.14–0.56
	D	535 mg	3–9	No	No	Yes	$0.12–0.36
3	E	520 mg	1–3 (with meals)	No	No	No	$0.21–0.63
	F	160 mg	2–3 (bedtime)	Yes (0.2%)	Yes (1)	Yes	$0.38–0.57
	G	530 mg	3 (bedtime)	Yes (0.1%)	No	Yes	$0.18
	H	100 mg	1–2 (bedtime)	Yes (0.8%)	No	Yes	$0.10–0.20
	I	?	2 (bedtime)	Yes (0.8%)	Yes (4)	No	$0.76
	J	?	2–6 as needed	No	Yes (4)	No	$0.46–1.38

nal properties are extracted from the rootstock. These constituents, particularly the essential oil, can be affected by handling, drying, storage, and processing of the root. For example, care should be taken in handling and processing the root so as to avoid damaging the cells containing the essential oil. Furthermore, excessive washing may substantially reduce the extractable content from the root. Recommendations have been made for a number of proper drying techniques to maximize preservation of the essential oil. Improper or protracted drying procedures bring about a chemical reaction that produces an unpleasant scent, compared with the faint but distinctive camphorlike smell that valerian should have.

Stability and Freshness

The stability of the different constituents in valerian varies over time and is affected by storage conditions. Valerian should be stored in closed containers and protected from light and moisture. While valerenic acid and its breakdown products are relatively stable, the valepotriates are more susceptible to degradation when stored at higher temperatures (greater than 40°C), greater humidity, and acid mediums (pH of less than 3), or with exposure to water. In fact, in analyses of commercial tinctures, valepotriates were undetectable after 60 days (Lutowski and Turowska, 1973; Bos et al., 1996). In contrast, the essential oil, which is generally considered to be more stable, degrades over time as well when in the powdered root form, by as much as 50 percent in six months in some cases. The most important criterion to look for is still appropriate standardization to valerenic acid—the best we can do with what we know at this time.

These issues raise concerns about the potency and shelf life of these products. Formal guidelines regarding the appropriate shelf life of valerian preparations have not been established, so expiration dates are not necessarily reliable. Nonetheless, it makes sense to reject any brand that has no expiration date at all. If the manufacturer does not know enough to put an expiration date on the package, it does not know that the product has a limited shelf life, which only makes you wonder what else this manufacturer is ignorant of.

A Few Consumer Tips

So how is a consumer to know what brands are good and which ones are not? Guidelines for things to consider when shopping for herbal products (or other dietary supplements for that matter) are listed in the Introduction. It can also be helpful to learn what brands other consumers are using. While high sales can reflect good advertising and do not necessarily equate with product effectiveness, good sales may be indicative of a product that works. So check to see what products appear to moving in the store and selling—Do the packages appear clean and fresh, or are they gathering dust and cobwebs?

Also look for the following indications of responsible, high-quality processing and packaging:

- A statement of product standardization to at least 0.5 percent of valerenic acid and of the dose per unit (i.e., mg/pill).
- Dosing recommendations that fit within the guidelines given in Table 21. In our survey, we found dosages ranging from one 100-mg (unspecified whether root or extract) pill one to two hours before bedtime to three 535-mg capsules (containing extract) three times a day as needed or three to six tablets at bedtime—doses not supported by findings from scientific studies!
- A complete listing of all ingredients. Compounds other than valerian that are in a preparation should be listed, including the amount in each recommended dose. You may find products with names that indicate that more than one ingredient is included but that fail to list those ingredients and their amounts on the label. It is always prudent to know the contents of the medicinal or supplemental products you ingest, so avoid products that fail to meet this criterion.

I tried a new brand of valerian and got headaches.
Am I developing some kind of problem with this herb?

Not necessarily. The problem may not be with valerian but with the brand you're now using. Different brands could vary in the side effects they produce, especially if your new product contains another ingredient. Check the label. If no additional ingredient is listed, try another brand with no extra ingredients listed to see if you have the same side effects with that one. There's also a chance that side effects may differ somewhat within a given product brand depending on the form selected (such as dried powdered extract vs. tincture), but this is not known to be a concern with valerian.

Can I buy valerian in large quantities to save money?

Beware of the "large economy size" package where valerian is concerned. As explained earlier, valerian and other herbs have limited shelf lives. The expiration date may be nearer than you would expect, and if there is none, that large bottle could cost you a lot of money in ineffective doses you shouldn't bother to take.

What does price variation among brands mean?

Not very much. A more expensive brand is not always a better brand. By paying a higher price, you may well be helping to pay for more costly advertising, fancy packaging, and the like. But lower prices are not always a bargain either. In the survey we conducted, we found the prices between brands of valerian varied from $3.57 for 100 capsules to $22.95 for 60 capsules (see Table 22). While brand D may appear less expensive at first glance, when you consider the number of pills recommended daily, it comes to $0.12–0.36 per day—which is actually in the middle of the cost range for all of the brands surveyed. What at first may appear to be a bargain may not always be the case! So, do not base your decision to buy an herbal product on the cost alone. Keep in mind the overall potency of the product too. One capsule of one brand may be all you need to get the same strength as three capsules of another brand.

When I opened the bottle of valerian I bought, I was hit by a wave of dirty sweat sock odor. Is that the way it's supposed to smell?

Older plant material or that which has been dried improperly is characteristically malodorous, an all-too-familiar aroma to valerian consumers. This unpleasant odor is attributable to the enzymatic breakdown of the valepotriates into isovaleric acid. In fact, one of the old names for valerian is "Phu." (Of note, an odor-controlled preparation has been developed and is available in Europe.) While the smell is most unpleasant, this is by no means an indication that the product has "spoiled" or is substandard. In fact, in ancient times, it was believed that the potency of the herb resided in the smell and that pleasant-smelling valerian was inactive.

Is Valerian Working for You?

I thought valerian wasn't supposed to give me a sleeping pill hangover, but I felt really fuzzy-headed the morning after I first tried it. What should I do?

Start by cutting the dose in half. If you find that this side effect does not subside cut the dose back further, and this side effect should resolve.

How can I tell if I'm getting what I should from valerian?

First, recall what your situation was like *before* beginning treatment. Were you having trouble falling asleep? Or were you tossing and turning, having difficulty staying asleep? How long did you sleep overall (remember—we all vary in the amount of sleep we need to feel refreshed)? Were you getting up in the morning unrested and worn out? Did you follow good sleep hygiene practices (see Table 18 for a list of sleep hygiene dos and don'ts)? Also, consider how you were feeling during the day. Other problems reported during the daytime by people with insomnia are noted in the section "When Should You Treat Insomnia?" (page 198).

Before trying valerian, consider these issues and make a list of the problems you are experiencing. Also, if you are not already doing so, take note of the sleep hygiene practices discussed earlier in this chapter and try to integrate these into your evening routine. With treatment over time, refer back to this list to see if valerian is helping and, if so, in which areas and how much. In doing this, you will have a better idea of how effective the treatment has been. You can also use a medication log like the one described in Chapter 1.

What if it seems like valerian isn't working for me?

If after three to four weeks or so of treatment with valerian at the doses recommended you have not noted improvement, you may need to increase the dose. If you are taking the maximum dose and there is no response, you may want to try another brand. You should also make sure you're practicing good sleep hygiene (see Table 18).

If the valerian is still not effective, it is possible that valerian simply is not strong enough for you and that some other sleeping medicine would help. It also may be time to consider the possibility that your sleep trouble is a sign of another problem altogether. Talk to your doctor.

Is there anything special I should do to stop taking valerian?

When taken as recommended, valerian can be discontinued with minimal discomfort. As with other hypnotics, you may note initial "rebound insomnia" immediately after discontinuation, but it will probably be mild and transient. There is no data to support a need to taper the dose prior to discontinuation.

What Lies Ahead?

While valerian has been used successfully for hundreds of years, we still have much to learn about it. Some of the important issues to consider and explore in the years to come include these potential uses:

- As a stress modulator in acutely stressful situations such as being in heavy traffic
- As a way to modulate extreme ongoing stress, such as that experienced by soldiers and refugees (remembering valerian's use for World War I veterans), or the more chronic effects seen afterward
- As a treatment for more pervasive anxiety states

It would also be desirable to see how valerian compares to the newer hypnotic drugs, specifically Ambien and Sonata. Finally, we will want to know how safe and effective valerian might be in treating sleep and anxiety in children.

ESSENTIAL FACTS ABOUT VALERIAN

Main Uses	Hypnotic (sleep aid)
Other Reported Uses	Anxiolytic (anti-anxiety), stress relief, possibly antidepressant
When Not to Use This Herb	Beyond six weeks of use; use caution in those under 18; while taking other psychoactive drugs (those affecting the brain and behavior), use under a physician's guidance
Side Effects	Mild headaches, nausea, nervousness, palpitations, morning grogginess; with longtime use of large doses, headache, excitability and mental agitation, restlessness, nausea and diarrhea, palpitations, and slowed reaction time with dulling of senses
When to Expect Positive Effects	For insomnia, after 30 to 90 minutes; full effect for insomnia or anxiety may take three to four weeks
Common Preparation Forms	Capsules, pills, liquid extracts, tinctures, infusions, teas
Average Effective Daily Dosage	300 to 600 mg, standardized to at least 0.5 percent valerenic acid, taken in one dose before bed for insomnia; in one to three divided doses for anxiety

Glossary

Acute   Referring to a symptom or disorder that arises rapidly.

Adaptogen   A remedy that restores functioning to normal. If the system is overactive, it slows down. If the system is underactive, it speeds up.

Addiction   A state of physical and psychological dependence produced by habitual use of certain drugs, with the core connotation of loss of control over use.

Allergy   Exaggerated physical response caused by a stimulus or substance to which the person has become hypersensitive from previous exposure.

Alterative   A substance that restores health.

Alternative medicine   What is not taught in medical schools nor covered by insurance; traditional health care systems and their components, typically involving spirituality, a "vital force," and holism (i.e., belief in a unity underlying all diversity)—these qualities seem to distinguish alternative medicine from conventional medicine.

Analgesic   A substance that reduces pain.

Antidepressant   A medication intended to alleviate the symptoms of depression.

Anti-inflammatory   Reducing inflammation by acting on body mechanisms without directly acting on the cause of inflammation; e.g., glucocorticoids, aspirin.

Antispasmodic   Preventing spasms.

Anxiety   A feeling of fear or danger; a distressing apprehension that something bad will occur.

Anxiolytic   A medication intended to alleviate the symptoms of anxiety.

Aphrodisiac   A substance that increases sexual desire.

Benzodiazepine   A class of drug frequently used to treat anxiety or insomnia (e.g., Valium, Librium, Serzone, Xanax, Klonopin, Ativan, Dalmane, Restoril).

Bitter   A bitter-tasting tonic that stimulates digestion or appetite.

Botanical   Of or relating to plants or to the scientific study of plant life.

Bud   An immature shoot, often covered by scales.

Calyx   The leafy part of a flower.

CAM   Complementary and alternative medicine. An umbrella term for all the approaches to medicine not included in traditional medicine of the modern West, from acupuncture to shiatsu to naturopathy to chiropractic to herbalism. As these treatments become more and more widely accepted, however, the term becomes less and less appropriate.

Carminative   A remedy that reduces gastrointestinal or bowel symptoms.

CBT   Cognitive-behavioral therapy, a form of psychotherapy that identifies a person's faulty thought patterns and works to replace them with healthier thought patterns.

Chronic   Long term, ongoing.

Clinical   Based on direct observation of a patient by a doctor, as in a diagnosis based on observation by the doctor.

Clinical trial   A research experiment using human subjects, whose response to the form of treatment being studied is observed, assessed, and recorded by doctors. Clinical trials can be of many different designs. They can occur during drug development for new drugs, as well as with established, marketed drugs. The best known type is the randomized double-blind placebo-controlled trial, where assignment to treatment is determined in a randomized way and not by the doctor's choice.

Cognitive   Related to thinking.

Commission E   The German government's regulatory body that investigates the efficacy and safety of herbal treatments and grants approval to them for specific uses. Commission E's findings have been published in the Commission E Monograph, which has served as the foundation for much research into herbal remedies in the rest of the world, including the United States.

Complementary and alternative medicine   *See* CAM.

Contraindication   A symptom, condition, other treatment, or other factor that would make a treatment inadvisable. For example, taking an MAOI drug would contraindicate the use of St. John's wort.

CRH Corticotropin-releasing hormone. A chemical produced in the hypothalamus of the brain.

Crossover study A comparison of two treatments, in which subjects receive one treatment and are then "crossed over" to receive the other.

Decoction A tea prepared by placing an herb in water and bringing it to a boil. Herb and liquid are then separated by straining, leaving the tea to drink.

Dementia A stable and progressive deterioration in cognitive functioning in the setting of a stable level of consciousness.

Dependence Physical or psychological dependence on a drug that when stopped abruptly leads to withdrawal symptoms.

Dietary supplement A product that is considered neither food nor drug, as specified under the Dietary Supplement Health and Education Act (*see* DSHEA). Most herbal remedies are categorized as dietary supplements for marketing purposes. The DSHEA forbids manufacturers of dietary supplements from making any claims that the supplement cures any disease, disorder, or other health problem but allows them to make claims about promotion of general well-being, such as "promotes central nervous system health" for St. John's wort.

Dietary supplements Vitamin, mineral, herb, or other botanical or amino acid.

Disorder An abnormal physical or mental condition.

Dopamine A neurochemical that is responsible for aspects of movement, drive, sexual response, craving, and mood.

Dose Amount of therapeutic substance to be taken during a specified time period, often expressed in milligrams (mg), milliliters (ml), or drops.

Double-blind, controlled study A clinical research study in which neither the patient nor the doctor knows who is taking the treatment being investigated and who is taking a placebo. These studies are important because they reduce the bias, or influence of expectation, that often occurs when one can identify the treatment.

DSHEA The 1994 Dietary Supplement Health and Education Act, passed to distinguish between drugs, which must undergo a lengthy, expensive testing process before approval by the FDA, and products such as vitamins and herbal remedies, which are prohibited from claiming ability to treat illness but may claim the ability to promote wellness. The DSHEA encouraged the manufacture and marketing of the herbal remedies that consumers were demanding in the 1990s by removing the burden of costly testing and approval procedures, but it has been criticized for imposing too little regulation on such products.

DSM The *Diagnostic and Statistical Manual of Mental Disorders*, published by the American Psychiatric Association with the aim of standardizing diagnostic criteria. The manual contains diagnostic criteria for established psychiatric disorders, including depression, anxiety, dementia, and other disorders discussed in this book. Its most recent edition, the fourth, was published in 1994.

Efficacy The effectiveness, or degree of change in symptoms, that a treatment brings. *See* also Potency.

Epilepsy Chronic seizure disorder, often associated with alteration of consciousness.

Essential oil Volatile terpene derivatives responsible for the odor or taste of a plant.

Expectorant A substance that increases bronchial secretion, enabling it to be coughed up.

Extract A concentrated form of an herb, obtained by treating the crude herb with an appropriate solvent (e.g., water, alcohol) and then removing most or all of the solvent; ranges from the mildest infusions and decoctions to tinctures, to liquid extracts, to solid extracts. A standardized extract is a product guaranteed to contain a standardized level of active constituents.

FDA The federal Food and Drug Administration, which sets safety standards for the manufacture and sale of foods and drugs (both prescription and over-the-counter). Any substance sold as a medicine—with claims that it can treat the symptoms of an illness—must be approved by the FDA before being placed on the market. Herbal remedies, as long as they claim only to promote some form of wellness (such as "may increase peripheral circulation, thus increasing blood flow . . . " for ginkgo or "mood enhancement" for St. John's wort) need not go through the lengthy drug-approval process to be sold in stores. Labels must, however, contain a disclaimer to this effect: "These statements have not been evaluated by the Food and Drug Administration. This product is not intended to diagnose, treat, cure, or prevent any disease."

FDCA The Food, Drug, and Cosmetics Act, which sets the standards for drug development and whose stipulations must be followed by the manufacturer before its product can receive FDA approval for the treatment of disease and consequently be marketed to the public.

Flavonoid   A general term for a group of flavone-containing compounds found widely in nature, including many compounds that make up the pigments that give plants their color.

Flower   The reproductive structure of flowering plants.

Fluid extract   Concentrated extract in which 1 ml is equivalent to 1 gram of the original botanical.

Folk medicine   Practices not stemming from or sanctioned by institutionalized medicine but based on a history of home or traditional use in a culture.

Fruit   The matured ovary of flowering plants, with or without accessory parts.

GABA   Gamma-aminobutyric acid. A brain neurotransmitter (chemical) related to control of anxiety.

Ginkgo biloba   The oldest tree species known on earth; ginkgo preparations are standardized from the whole-leaf extract.

Hallucination   Visual, auditory, tactile, or olfactory perception of objects that are not actually present.

Herb   A plant with a nonwoody stem that dies back in the winter.

Herbal   Referring to any part of a plant that has value as food, fragrance, or medicine. An herbal remedy may come from the flowers, leaves, seeds, stems, or roots of any plant, including trees.

Holistic   Referring to the theory of the universe that treats everything as whole systems rather than as individual parts; in medicine, referring to a diagnostic and treatment approach that takes into account the whole body, including the mind. It can include all types of treatment, whether herbal, antibiotic, chiropractic, or whatever.

Homeopathic   A product containing very small or no material doses of a substance that would, in normal doses, cause symptoms of the disease that it is intended to treat.

Homeopathy   The practice of treating symptoms with a very tiny dose of a substance that would normally produce those symptoms. Plant-derived remedies are often used in homeopathy (e.g., *Hypericum perforatum* [St. John's wort]; pulsatilla). The substance used to treat the symptoms in a sick person is the same that induces those symptoms when given to a healthy person. Homeopathy is controversial because of its assertion that the less of the original substance there is, the more potent the medicine becomes.

Hyperforin   One of the chemical components of St. John's wort that is now thought to be responsible for the herb's antidepressant effects (*see* Hypericin). A few St. John's wort preparations are standardized for hyperforin.

Hypericin   The chemical component of St. John's wort initially believed to be the sole source of its antidepressant effects (*see* Hyperforin). Most St. John's wort preparations are standardized for hypericin.

Hypericum   A genus containing approximately 300 species, of which St. John's wort (*Hypericum perforatum*) is one.

Hypnotic   A drug or herb that induces sleep; synonymous with *soporific*.

Hypothyroidism   Reduced production of thyroid hormone, which produce symptoms of depression.

In vitro   Literally, "in glass," referring to experiments done in an artificial environment rather than within a living body (*see* In vivo). Because they do not duplicate the workings of a human or other body, such experiments yield hints about mechanisms of action but do not prove that a treatment will have the same effect in a living being.

In vivo   Literally, "in the living," referring to experiments that use live people or animals. *In vivo* experiments done on human beings are considered more reliably indicative of how a treatment will work in a person (*see* In vitro).

Interaction   The effect that may take place in the human body between two drugs, a drug and an herb, a drug or herb and a food or other environmental condition. Knowing what factors may interact with herbal remedies is important for their safe use.

Interleukin-6   A chemical present in the body that is related to the immune response and that may be important in depression.

Kavalactone   One of the chemical compounds contained in kava, six of which are known to be the active anxiety-reducing components of the herb. Also called *kavapyrone*. Kava products should be standardized for kavalactones.

Kavapyrone   *See* Kavalactone.

Limbic system   Brain structures, including hippocampus, dentate gyrus, and amygdala, that are associated with emotions.

Maceration   Herb preparation softened by soaking.

MAO   Monoamine oxidase. An enzyme in the body that breaks down dopamine, noradrenaline (norepinephrine), and serotonin. MAO inhibitor drugs increase levels of these substances and help treat depression and anxiety.

Menopause   Permanent cessation of menstruation.

Meta-analysis   A statistical technique used when pooling together the results of many different studies.

Metabolite   Any product (foodstuff, intermediate, waste product) of metabolism.

Monoamine oxidase   *See* MAO.

Monograph   An in-depth written report on one subject, such as the reports in the Commission E Monograph on herbal remedies.

Mood stabilizer   A class of drugs used to treat the manic symptoms of bipolar disorder (aka manic depression).

Neurochemical   A chemical in the brain or nervous system that transmits information (or a "message") from one nerve to another; synonymous with *neurotransmitter.*

Neuroleptic   A class of drug that is effective in treating schizophrenia.

Neurotoxic   Poisonous to the nerves.

Neurotransmitter   A chemical in the brain or nervous system that transmits information (or a "message") from one nerve to another; synonymous with *neurochemical.*

Noradrenaline   A neurotransmitter relevant to mood, anxiety, memory, and the alarm response; also called *norepinephrine.*

Ointment   A form of medicine used as an external application to the skin.

Oral   By mouth.

Placebo   An inactive substance used in a controlled study to verify findings about the active substance being studied through comparison. In a controlled study, one group of participants will be given the active substance and another group a placebo. Studies that only compare one medication to another (e.g., St. John's wort to Prozac) do not eliminate the possibility that one of the medications has merely had a "placebo effect"—the mysterious but common response that people have to inactive ingredients. When a placebo is given to a control group without the doctor or subject knowing which medicine they receive (*see* Double-blind controlled study), any response to the active ingredient can be viewed as more reliable.

Positive effect   The effect desired from a medicine or other treatment, such as the reduction of stress with the use of kava.

Potency   The amount of a medication that is needed to produce a given effect (*see* Efficacy).

Poultice   A therapeutic preparation made by the moistening of botanicals with oil or water, usually applied hot to the skin.

Prodromal   A precursor symptom to a disease—the early signs that a disorder, such as depression, may be beginning.

Psychogenic   Of psychological origin.

Resin   An amorphous brittle substance consisting of the hardened secretion of various plants, typically derived from the oxidation of terpenes.

Reuptake   The process by which a neurotransmitter is taken back up from the nerve synapse into the nerve cell and inactivated.

Rhizome   In botany, an underground stem.

Roborant   A strengthening agent, tonic.

Root   The anchoring part of the plant that also absorbs nutrients.

SAMe   S-Adenosylmethionine. A substance present in the body and available as a natural remedy to improve mood.

Secretagogue   A substance that increases secretion.

Sedative   A drug that sedates.

Serotonergic   A substance that has serotonin effects.

Serotonin   A chemical found throughout the body, relevant to mood, sleep, appetite, sex, and temperature regulation.

Side effect   Any effect outside the desired positive effect of a medicine. In general, side effects are those effects of a drug that are unwanted (e.g., nausea, sexual difficulty, weight gain), but they can sometimes be used to the advantage of the patient (e.g., an antidepressant drug that sedates as a side effect can be given at night to treat insomnia).

Soporific   A medicine that induces sleep. *See* Hypnotic.

SSRIs   Selective serotonin reuptake inhibitors, the newer generation of antidepressants. SSRIs inhibit reuptake(or "inactivation") of serotonin. They are safer and have fewer side effects than older antidepressants.

Standardization   The manufacturing process whereby a set amount of the active extract of an herb exists in a certain amount of the preparation by weight. Knowing how much substance is present can sometimes inform you if you are receiving enough of the active medicine, as well as assuring you that quantity does not vary from pill to pill.

Standardized extract   A process that results in a certain ingredient, or ingredients, of the herb being present at a known and constant amount in the product. (The standardized ingredient may or may not be the active, or medicinal, part of the plant.)

Stem   A supporting and conducting organ of the plant.

Subclinical   A condition that may be a partial manifestation of a disorder; it does not fit all of the diagnostic criteria for the disorder. Many people today use self-treatment with herbs to ameliorate the milder forms of depression, anxiety, and other disorders that are not as severe, as frequent, or as impairing as the full clinical disorder, for example, as described in *DSM-IV* (*see* DSM).

Sunburn   Reddening of the skin, with or without blistering, caused by exposure to ultraviolet light.

Synergism   When the combined effect of two or more substances is greater than their individual effects.

Syrup   A liquid preparation of medicinal substances in a concentrated aqueous solution of sucrose.

Taper   To cut down gradually on the dosage of a medicine so as to prevent any relapse, rebound, or other ill effects of sudden cessation of the medicine. Many herbal remedies do not appear to require tapering.

TCM   Traditional Chinese medicine. An integrated system of medicine used in China for over 2,000 years, which includes herbalism, acupuncture, diet, and exercise.

Tea   An infusion made by pouring boiling water over plant material and allowing it to steep for a period of time.

Tea, herbal   An herbal remedy made by an infusion of the active parts of the herb (such as the leaves) in hot water; herbal teas are generally thought to be less potent and usually require a much greater amount of the herb per dose.

Teratogenicity   Property of a drug that results in physical defects in the developing embryo.

Therapy   Any treatment for a health problem.

Tincture   An alcohol or water–alcohol solution. Glycerine can be used and produces a weaker, alcohol-free tincture.

Tincture   The liquid that results when an herbal extract is soaked in water or alcohol and the extract is then pressed; usually weaker and less economical than other forms; generally should be avoided by anyone with alcohol problems since most tinctures use alcohol as the solvent, but sometimes believed to act more quickly than other forms.

Tolerance   Wearing off of the effects of a substance over time.

Tonic   A remedy that supposedly increases energy or strength.

Topical   A substance applied to the skin.

Traditional medicine   Can refer either to treatments that are conventionally used in medicine (e.g., current tradition) or medical approaches that have been used for a long time (i.e., rooted in cultural tradition) and that are usually outside of current conventional practice.

Tranquilizer   A drug that calms an anxious, agitated, or restless person.

Tricyclic antidepressant   A three-ring-structure antidepressant, widely used before the SSRIs. They are effective but have many side effects.

Valepotriate   One of the active ingredients in valerian believed to play a role in its sleep-promoting qualities but also suspected to have some toxicity when ingested in large quantities.

Valerenic acid   One of the active ingredients in valerian believed to be responsible for its sleep-promoting qualities and to which most valerian preparations are standardized

Volatile oil   Easily evaporated terpene derivatives found in plants that impart taste and aroma.

Withdrawal   Appearance of symptoms during the removal (withdrawal) of a drug. Symptoms may be similar to the underlying disorder or related to the drug's action on the body.

Resources

AUTHORITATIVE HERBAL TEXTS

Blumenthal, M., Klein, S., Busse, W. R., et al. *The Complete German Commission E Monographs: Therapeutic Guide to Herbal Medicines*. Newton, MA: Integrative Medicine Communication. 1998.

Translated from the original German monographs, this text provides authoritative information on the safety and efficacy of herbs and phytomedicinals, with a wealth of extra data.

British Herbal Medicine Association. *British Herbal Pharmacopoeia*. 1996.

Monographs covering identification and standards for plant material used in herbal products.

Miller, L. G., and Murray, W. J. *Herbal Medicinals: A Clinician's Guide*. Binghamton, NY: Haworth Press. 1998.

A case-based approach to herbal medicine to guide practitioners that provides information about herbal remedies and their interactions with conventional medicines.

Leung, A. Y., and Foster, S. *Encyclopedia of Common Natural Ingredients Used in Food, Drugs, and Cosmetics*. New York: Wiley. 1996.

Invaluable research resource for those involved in the manufacture and research of natural products.

PDR for Herbal Medicines. Montvale, NJ: Medical Economics Company. 1998.

Authoritative information from the company that produces the *Physicians' Desk Reference*.

Rosenthal, N. *St. John's Wort: The Herbal Way to Feeling Good*. New York: HarperCollins. 1998.

Schulz, V., Hänsel, R; and Tyler, V. E. *Rational Phytotherapy: A Physician's Guide to Herbal Medicine*, 3rd ed., 1st English ed. Translated by Terry C. Telger. New York: Springer-Verlag. 1998.

Scholarly guide to herbal medicine for physicians.

Tyler, V. E. *Tyler's Herbs of Choice: the Therapeutic Use of Phytomedicinals*. Binghamton, NY: Haworth Press. 1999.

Practical information on the traditional uses of herbal medicinals, active constituents, and clinical applications—partly anecdotal, primarily scientific.

Wichtl, M. *Herbal Drugs and Phytopharmaceuticals*. Translated by Norman Bisset. Stuttgart, Germany: MedPharm GmbH Scientific Publishers. 1994.

References pharmacopeial monographs, sources, synonyms, constituent indications, side effects, preparation of tea, commercially available phytomedicines, regulatory status, authentication using macroscopic, microscopic, and chromatographic techniques. 181 detailed monographs. Color prints of the dried part and whole plant in natural habitat.

JOURNALS

Alternative Therapies in Health and Medicine
Website: www.alternative.therapies.com

A journal that provides a forum for sharing information concerning the practical use of alternative therapies in preventing and treating disease, healing illness, and promoting health. The journal encourages the integration of alternative therapies with conventional medical practices in a way that provides for a rational, individualized, comprehensive approach to health care.

HerbalGram
Website: www.herbalgram.com

The journal of the American Botanical Council and the Herb Research Foundation. A full-color quarterly publication with peer-reviewed scientific articles, herb news and market data, and discussion of regulatory and legal issues. The mail-order book department offers a wide selection of books on herbal topics. This is an informative publication for professionals and the general public.

Journal of Alternative and Complementary Medicine
Website: www.liebertpub.com

A bimonthly journal that includes observational and analytical reports on treatments outside the realm of allopathic medicine that are gaining interest and warranting research to assess their therapeutic value.

Medical Herbalism
Website: www.medherb.com

An online newsletter for clinical practitioners, written by Paul Bergner, researcher, writer, and educator at the Rocky Mountain Center for Botanical Studies, Boulder, Colorado. The journal site also puts out a listing of schools of herbal medicine.

GOVERNMENT RESOURCES

European Agency for the Evaluation of Medicinal Products
7 Westferry Circus
Canary Wharf
London E14 4HB, United Kingdom
Tel: 44 (0) 171 418 8400
Website: www.edura.org/emea.html

The EAEMA serves as the focal point for the new European system of authorizing medicinal products for human and veterinary use, which is designed to promote public health and the free circulation of pharmaceuticals.

Food and Drug Administration
HFI-40
Rockville, MD 20857
Tel: (888) INFO-FDA
Website: www.fda.gov

The U.S. regulatory body that protects public health by ensuring the safety of food (including dietary supplements), cosmetics, medicines, and medical devices in humans and food and drugs in animals.

National Institutes of Health, National Center for Complimentary
and Alternative Medicine (NCCAM)
Website: nccam.nih.gov

The National Institutes of Health (Bethesda, MD) maintains this site. Complementary and Alternative Medicine Citation Index (website: http://altmed.od.nih.gov/nccam/resources/cam-ci)

From the National Library of Medicine's MEDLINE database.

Public Information Clearinghouse
P.O. Box 8218
Silver Spring, MD 20907-8218
Tel: (888) 644-6226
Fax: (301) 495-4957

Website: nccam.nih.gov/nccam/fcp/clearinghouse/
A good source for fact sheets and information with government clearance.

National Library of Medicine
PubMed
Website: www.ncbi.nlm.nih.gov/entrez/query.fcgi?db=pubmed
Free public access to the National Library of Medicine MEDLINE database of clinical research is now available on the World Wide Web. Searching the 9 million citations in the MEDLINE database on the World Wide Web is simple and rapid with PubMed and its Related Articles feature. High-quality research resources are accessible to all.

Office of Dietary Supplements
National Institutes of Health
Building 31, Room 1B25
31 Center Drive, MSC 2086
Bethesda, MD 20892-2086
Tel: (301) 435-2920
Fax: (301) 480-1845
Email: ods@nih.gov
Website: dietary-supplements.info.nih.gov
A congressionally mandated office within the National Institutes of Health, the Office of Dietary Supplements supports research and disseminates research results in the area of dietary supplements. At their website, they maintain the IBIDS Dietary Supplements References Database, which contains more than 325,000 scientific abstracts and citations about dietary supplements.

MENTAL HEALTH ORGANIZATIONS

Alzheimer's Association
919 North Michigan Avenue, Suite 1000
Chicago, IL 60611-1676
Tel: (800) 272-3900; (312) 335-8700
Fax: (312) 335-1110
Email: info@alz.org
Website: www.alz.org
Provides information, support, and assistance on issues related to Alzheimer's disease.

Alzheimer's Disease Education and Referral Center
P.O. Box 8250
Silver Spring, MD 20907-8250

Tel: (800) 438-4380
Email: adear@alzheimers.org
Website: www.alzheimers.org

A service of the National Institute of Aging (NIA), part of the National Institutes of Health. The center provides information about Alzheimer's disease, its impact on families and health professionals, and research into possible causes and cures.

Anxiety Disorders Association of America (ADAA)
11900 Parklawn Drive
Rockville, MD 20852-2624
Tel: (301) 231-9350
Website: www.adaa.org

An organization of mental health professionals and consumers interested in the prevention and cure of anxiety disorders and improving the lives of those who suffer from them.

American Psychiatric Association
1400 K Street, NW
Washington, DC 20005-2492
Tel: (202) 682-6000
Website: www.psych.org

A medical specialty society of health care providers who specialize in the diagnosis and treatment of mental and emotional illnesses and substance use disorders.

American Psychological Association
750 First Street, NE
Washington, DC 20002-4242
Tel: (202) 336-5500
Website: www.apa.org

A professional organization of researchers, educators, clinicians, consultants, and students that works to advance psychology as a science, as a profession, and as a means of promoting human welfare.

National Alliance for the Mentally Ill
Colonial Place Three
2107 Wilson Blvd., Suite 300
Arlington, VA 22201-3042
Tel: (800) 950-6264
Website: www.nami.org

Provides support to persons with severe mental illness and their family members and promotes advocacy, research, and educational activities.

National Depression and Manic Depressive Association
730 North Franklin Street, Suite 501
Chicago, IL 60610-3526
Tel: (800) 826-3632
Fax: (312) 642-7243
Email: myrtis@aol.com
Website: www.ndmda.org

An advocacy organization for patients, families, professionals, and the public that provides education, fosters self-help, strives to improve access to care and to advocate for research in the treatment of depressive and manic–depressive illnesses.

National Sleep Foundation
1522 K Street, NW, Suite 500
Washington, DC 20005
Website: www.sleepfoundation.org

A nonprofit organization that promotes public understanding of sleep and sleep disorders and supports related education, research, and advocacy to improve public health and sleep.

Royal College of Psychiatrists
17 Belgrave Square
London SW1X 8PG, United Kingdom
Tel: 44 (0) 171 235 2351
Website: www.rcpsych.ac.uk/index.htm

A professional and educational body for psychiatrists in the United Kingdom and the Republic of Ireland that works to advance and promote the science, research, education, and practice of psychiatry and related subjects.

HERB-RELATED ORGANIZATIONS AND PROFESSIONAL SOCIETIES

Herb-Related Organizations

Alternative Medicine Foundation
5411 W. Cedar Lane, Suite 205-A
Bethesda, MD 20814
Tel: (301) 581-0116
Website: www.amfoundation.org

A nonprofit organization providing educational resources to the public and professionals about alternative systems of health care, treatment, and diagnosis.

American Botanical Council (ABC)
P.O. Box 144345
Austin, TX 78714-4345
Tel: (512) 926-4900
Fax: (512) 926-2345
Website: www.herbalgram.org
 A scientific research and education organization; publisher of *HerbalGram* and other education information, and an extensive book catalog.

American Herb Association (AHA)
P.O. Box 1673
Nevada City, CA 95959
Tel: (530) 265-9552
Fax: (530) 274-3140
 Publishes quarterly newsletter.

American Herbal Pharmacopoeia (AHP)
P.O. Box 5159
Santa Cruz, CA 95063
Tel: (831) 461-6317
Fax: (831) 475-6219
Website: www.herbal-ahp.org
 Publishes extensive monographs on leading herbs.

American Herbalists Guild
P.O. Box 70
Roosevelt, UT 84066
Tel: (435) 722-8434
Website: www.healthy.net/herbalists
 Founded in 1989, this nonprofit, educational organization represents the goals and voices of herbalists and promotes and maintains excellence in herbalism. Membership consists of professionals, general members, and benefactors.

European Scientific Cooperative on Phytotherapy (ESCOP)
Argyle House, Gandy Street
Exeter, Devon EX4 3LS, United Kingdom
Tel: 011 (44-1392) 424-626
Fax: 011 (44-1392)424-864
Website: info.exeter.ac.uk/phytonet
 European group producing therapeutic monographs and *The European Phytojournal.*

Herb Research Foundation (HRF)
1007 Pearl Street, Suite 200
Boulder, CO 80302
Tel: (800) 748-2617
Fax: (303) 449-7849
Website: www.herbs.org
    Provides custom literature reviews, toll-free line for consumer information; *HerbalGram* for members.

Herb Society
Deddington Hill Farm
Warmington
Banbury OX17 1XB, United Kingdom
Tel: 44 (0) 129 569 2000
Website: dspace.dial.pipex.com/herbsociety
    The Herb Society is an educational charity dedicated to the dissemination of knowledge about the healing properties of herbs and their use in the community, as well as to the support of further research in the healing properties of herbs.

Herb Society of America
9019 Kirtland Chardon Road
Kirtland, OH 44094
Tel: (440) 256-0514
Website: www.herbsociety.org
    The society was founded in 1933 for the purpose of furthering the knowledge and use of herbs.

U.S. Pharmacopeia (USP)
12601 Twinbrook Parkway
Rockville, MD 20852
Tel: (800) 822-8772; international: +1 (301) 881-0666
Website: www.usp.org
    In its mission to promote public health, the USP establishes standards to ensure the quality of medicines for both human and veterinary uses and develops authoritative information about the appropriate use of medicines.

Professional Societies

American Association of Naturopathic Physicians (AANP)
601 Valley Street, Suite 105
Seattle, WA 98109
Tel: (206) 298-0126

Website: www.naturopathic.org
A professional organization of naturopathic doctors who have graduated from an accredited four-year postgraduate school.

American Association of Oriental Medicine (AAOM)
433 Front Street
Catasauqua, PA 18032-2506
Tel: (888) 500-7999
Website: www.aaom.org
A professional organization of acupuncturists and practitioners of Oriental medicine.

American Herbalists Guild (AHG)
P.O. Box 70
Roosevelt, UT 84066
Tel: (435) 722-8434
Website: www.healthy.net/herbalists/
A professional society of herbalists.

British Herbal Medical Association
Website: info.ex.ac.uk/phytonet/bhma.html
Founded in 1964 to advance the science and practice of herbal medicine in the United Kingdom, including publication of the *British Herbal Pharmacopoeia* and *British Herbal Compendium* (Vol. 1). The membership of this organization includes companies manufacturing herbals, practitioners, academicians, pharmacists, students of phytotherapy, and others.

European Herbal Practitioners Association
Website: www.users.globalnet.co.uk/~epha
This organization works to foster unity within the herbal profession, to promote the availability of professional herbal treatment, and to raise the standards of training and practice within the profession. Members include the main professional herbal practitioner associations in the United Kingdom and other parts of Europe.

Faculty of Homeopathy
15 Clerkenwell Close
London EC1R 0AA, United Kingdom
Tel: 44 (0) 171 566 7810
A society promoting the scientific development of homeopathy and regulating the education, training, and practice of homeopathy by all statutorily registered health care professionals.

National Center for Homeopathy
801 North Fairfax St., Suite 306
Alexandria, VA 22314
Tel: (703) 548-7790
   Information resource on American homeopathy; list of practitioners.

National Institute of Medical Herbalists
56 Longbrook Street
Exeter, Devon EX4 6AH, United Kingdom
Tel: 44 (0) 139 242 6022
Website: www.btinterenet.com/~nimh
   The United Kingdom's leading professional organization of practitioners of
herbal medicine.

OTHER HELPFUL WEBSITES

Fact Sheets on Alternative Medicine
Website: cpmcnet.columbia.edu/dept/rosenthal/Databases.html
   The Richard and Hinda Rosenthal Center for Complementary and Alternative Medicine at Columbia University Medical Center, New York, NY, offers information on established worldwide resources on alternative medicine to facilitate research by both professionals and the public.

Mental Health Net
Website: www.mentalhelp.net
   An online mental health directory and guide, providing information about
disorders, treatments, and professional resources, as well as a reading room.

MentalHealth Infosource
Website: www.mhsource.com
   An online resource offering a wide range of educational and other informa-
tional resources and links.

World Health Organization (WHO)
Avenue Appia 20
1211 Geneva 27, Switzerland
Tel: 011 (41 22) 791-2111
Fax: 011 (41 22) 791-3111
Website: www.who.org
   International body dealing with global health issues.

References

GENERAL

American Psychiatric Association. *Diagnostic and Statistical Manual of Mental Disorders*. 4th ed. Washington, DC: American Psychiatric Association, 1994.

Blumenthal M, Goldberg A, Hall T, et al. *Commission E Monographs*. Austin, TX: American Herbal Council, 1998.

Blumenthal M, Klein S, Busse WR, et al. *The Commission E Monographs*. Newton, MA: Integrative Medicine Communications, 1998.

Brown D. *Herbal Prescriptions for Better Health*. Rocklin, CA: Prima Publishing, 1996.

Howard M. *Traditional Folk Remedies: A Comprehensive Herbal*. London: Century, 1987.

Murray MT. *The Healing Power of Herbs*. 2nd ed. Rocklin, CA: Prima Publishing, 1995.

Newall CA, Anderson LA, Phillipson JD. *Herbal Medicines: A Guide for Health-Care Professionals*. London: Pharmaceutical Press, 1996.

Schultz V, Hansel R, Tyler VE. *Rational Phytotherapy: A Physician's Guide to Herbal Medicine*. 3rd ed. Berlin: Springer, 1998.

Styron W. *Darkness Visible: A Memoir of Madness*. New York: Random House, 1990.

CHAPTER 1. St. John's Wort: The Herb Of Light

Biber A, Fischer H, Röaner A, et al. Oral bioavailability of hyperforin from hypericum extracts in rats and human volunteers. *Pharmacopsychiatry*, 1998, *31*, 36–43.

Bloomfield H. *Healing Anxiety with Herbs.* New York: HarperCollins, 1998.

Bloomfield HH, Nordfors M, McWilliams P. *Hypericum and Depression.* Los Angeles, CA: Prelude Press, 1996.

Cass H. *St. John's Wort: Nature's Blues Buster.* Garden City, NY: Avery, 1997.

Chatterjee SS, Nöldner M, Kode E, et al. Antidepressant activity of hypericum perforatum and hyperforin: The neglected possibility. *Pharmacopsychiatry,* 1998, *31,* 7–15.

Connor KM, Vaughan DS. *Kava: Nature's Stress Relief.* New York: Avon Books, 1999.

Cooper W, James J. An observational study of the safety and efficacy of hypericin in HIV and subjects. *International Conference in AIDS,* 1990, *6,* 369 (Abstract 2063).

Czekalla J, Gastpar M, Hübner W-D, et al. The effect of hypericum extract on cardiac conduction as seen in the electrocardiogram compared to that of imipramine. *Pharmacopsychiatry,* 1997, *30,* 86–88.

DeSmet PAGM, Nolen WA. St. John's wort as an antidepressant. *British Medical Journal,* 1996, *313,* 241–242.

Dressing H, Köhler S, Muller WE. Improvement of sleep quality with a highly dosed valerian/balm preparation. *Psychopharmacotherapie,* 1996, *3,* 123–130.

Ernst E. Second thoughts about safety of St. John's wort. *Lancet,* 1999, *354,* 2014–2016.

Eysenck HJ. *Manual of the Maudsley Personality Inventory.* London: University of London Press, 1969.

Hall, SS. Fear itself. *New York Times Magazine,* Feb. 28, 1999.

Hamilton M. The assessment of anxiety states by rating. *British Journal of Medical Psychology,* 1959, *32,* 50–55.

Hamilton M. Development of a rating scale for primary depressive illness. *British Journal of Clinical Psychology,* 1967, *6,* 278–296.

Hänsgen KD, Vesper J. Antidepressant efficiency of a high dose hypericum extract [In German]. *Münchener Mediziniscle Wochenschrift,* 1996, *138,* 29/35–33/39.

Hänsgen KD, Vesper J, Ploch M. Multicenter double-blind study examining the antidepressant effectiveness of the hypericum extract LI160. *Journal of Geriatric Psychiatry and Neurology,* 1994, *7*(Suppl. 1), S15–8.

Hocart C, Frankhauser B, Buckle D. Chemical archaeology of kava, a potent brew. *Rapid Communication in Mass Spectrometry,* 1993, *7,* 219–224.

Holmes TH, Rahe RH. The Social Readjustment Rating Scale. *Journal of Psychosomatic Research,* 1967, *11,* 213-218.

Kasper S. Treatment of seasonal affective disorder (SAD) with hypericum extract. *Pharmacopsychiatry,* 1997, *30*(Suppl. 2), 89–93.

Kramer PD. *Listening to Prozac.* New York: Penguin Books, 1993.

Lebot V, Merlin M, Lindstrom L. *The Pacific Elixir.* Rochester, VT: Healing Arts Press, 1997.

Linde K, Ramirez G, Mulrow CD, et al. St. John's wort for depression: An overview and meta-analysis of randomized clinical trials. *British Medical Journal*, 1996, 313, 253–258.

Meruelo D, Lavie G, Lavie D. Therapeutic agents with dramatic antiretroviral activity and little toxicity at effective doses: Aromatic polycyclic diones hypericin and pseudohypericin. *Proceedings of the National Academy of Sciences*, 1988, 85, 5230–5234.

Metcalfe M. The personality of depressive patients. In *Recent Developments in Affective Disorders*. Eds. A. Cooper and A. Walk. Ashford, England: Royal Medico-Psychological Association/Headley Books. 1968, 97–104.

Parker G. On brightening up: Triggers and trajectories to recovery from depression. *British Journal of Psychiatry*, 1996, 168, 263–264.

Philipp M, Kohnen R, Hiller K-O. Hypericum extract versus imipramine or placebo in patients with moderate depression: Randomized multicenter study of treatment for eight weeks. *British Medical Journal*, 1999, 319, 1534–1539.

Rosenthal N. *St. John's Wort: The Herbal Way to Feeling Good*. New York: HarperCollins, 1998.

Rosenthal N. *Winter Blues: Seasonal Affective Disorder: What It Is and How to Overcome It*. New York: Guilford, 1998.

Schellenberg R, Sauer S, Dimpfel W. Pharmacodynamic effects of two different hypericin extracts in health volunteers measured by quantitative EEG. *Pharmacopsychiatry*, 1998, 31, 44–53.

Shear MK, Otto MW, Pollack MH. *Structured interview guide for the Hamilton Anxiety Rating Scale*. Unpublished manuscript, University of Pittsburgh, Department of Psychiatry, 1998.

Staffkeldt B, Kert R, Brockmöller J, et al. Pharmacokinetics of hypericin and pseudohypericin after oral intake of the *Hypericum perforatum* extract LI160 in health volunteers. *Journal of Geriatric Psychiatry and Neurology*, 1994, 7(Suppl. 1), 47–53.

Stenbeck-Klose A, Wernet P. Successful long-term treatment over 40 months of HIV patients with intravenous hypericin. *International Conference on AIDS*, 1990, 9, 470 (Abstract 2012).

Thase ME, Laredo EE. *St. John's Wort: Nature's Mood Booster*. New York: Avon Books, 1998.

Vorbach EU, Arnold TKH, Hübner W-D. Efficacy and safety of St. John's wort extract LI-160 versus imipramine in patients with severe depressive episodes according to ICD-10. *Pharmacopsychiatry*, 1997, 30(Suppl. 2), 81–85.

Wheatley D. LI-160, an extract of St. John's wort, versus amitriptyline in mildly to moderately depressed outpatients: A controlled 6 week clinical trial. *Pharmacopsychiatry*, 1997, 30(Suppl. 2), 77–80.

Woelk H, Burkhard G, Grünwald J. Benefits and risks of the hypericum extract LI160: Drug monitoring study with 3250 patients. *Journal of Geriatric Psychiatry and Neurology*, 1994, 7(Suppl. 1), 34–38.

CHAPTER 2. Kava:
Tranquility from Paradise

Bloomfield HH. *Healing Anxiety with Herbs.* New York: HarperCollins, 1998.

Connor KM, Vaughan DS. *Kava: Nature's Stress Relief.* New York: Avon Books, 1999.

Davidson JR, Hughes DC, George LK, et al. The boundary of social phobia: Exploring the threshold. *Archives of General Psychiatry*, 1994, *51*(12), 975–983.

Davidson JRT, Hughes DL, George LK, et al. The epidemiology of social phobia: Findings from the Duke Epidemiological Catchment Area Study. *Psychological Medicine*, 1993, *23*, 709–718.

Dressing H, Kohler S, Müller WE. Improvement of sleep quality with a high-dose valerian/lemon balm preparation. *Psychopharmacotherapie*, 1996, *3*, 123–130.

Eisenberg DM, Davis RB, Ettner SL, et al. Trends in alternative medicine use in the United States, 1990–1997: Results of a follow-up national survey. *Journal of the American Medical Association*, 1998, *280*(18), 1569–1575.

Hamilton M. The assessment of anxiety states by rating. *British Journal of the Medical Psychology*, 1959, *32*, 50–55.

Herberg KW. Zum Einfluss von Kava-Spezialextrakt in kombination mit Ethylalkohol anf sicherheitsrelevante Leistunger [Effect of kava-special extract WS 1490 combined with ethyl alcohol on safety-relevant performance parameters]. *Blutalkohol*, 1993, *30*(20), 96–105.

Hocart C, Frankhauser B, Buckle D. Chemical archaeology of kava, a potent brew. *Rapid Communications in Mass Spectronomy*, 1993, *7*, 219–224.

Holmes TH, Rahe RH. The Social Readjustment Rating Scale. *Journal of Psychosomatic Research*, 1967, *11*, 213–218.

http://www.silk.net/personal/scombs/guide/html [Star Combs' Kava in Vanautu Webpage.]

http://www.theherbalist.com/kavakava.htm

Lebot V, Merlin M, Lindstrom L. *The Pacific Elixir.* Rochester, VT: Healing Arts Press, 1997.

Lehmann E, Kinzler E, Friedemann J. Efficacy of a special kava extract (*Piper methysticum*) in patients with states of anxiety, tension, and excitedness of non-mental origin. A double-blind placebo-controlled study of four weeks' treatment. *Phytomedicine*, 1996, *2*, 113–119.

Lindenberg D, Pitule-Schodel H. D,L-kavain in comparison with oxazepam in anxiety disorders: A double-blind study of clinical effectiveness [In German]. *Fortschritte der Medizin*, 1990, *108*(2), 49–50, 53–54.

Münte TF, Heinze HJ, Matzke M, et al. Effects of oxazepam and an extract of kava roots (Piper methysticum) on event-related potentials in a word recognition task. *Neuropsychobiology*, 1993, *27*, 46–53.

Sahelian R. *Kava: Nature's Answer to Anxiety*. Green Bay, WI: IMPAKT Communications, 1997.

Shear MK, Otto MW, Pollack MH. *Structured interview guide for the Hamilton Anxiety Rating Scale*. Unpublished manuscript, University of Pittsburgh, Department of Psychiatry, 1998.

Singh NN, Ellis CE, Singh YN. *A double-blind, placebo-controlled study of the effects of kava (Kavatrol™) on daily stress and anxiety in adults*. Paper presented at the 3rd Annual Alternative Therapies Symposium, San Diego, CA, April 1–4, 1998.

Stephen SHL. Fear itself. *New York Times Sunday Magazine*, Feb. 28, 1999.

Volz H-P, Kieser M. Kava-kava extract WS 1490 versus placebo in anxiety disorders: A randomized placebo-controlled 25-week outpatient trial. *Pharmacopsychiatry*, 1997, *30*, 1–5.

Warnecke G. Psychosomatische dysfunction en im weiblichen klimakterium: Klinishe wirksamkeit und vertraglichkeit van kava-extract WS 1490. *Fortschritte der Medizin*, 1991, *109*, 119–122.

Woelke H. Behandlung von angst-patienten. Kava-spezialextrakt WS -1490 bei angst-patientn in vergleich zu den benzodiazepines oxazepam und bromazepameine Doppelblindstudie in ärtzlichen Praxen. *Zeitschrift für Allgemeinmedizin*, 1993, *63*, 271–277.

CHAPTER 3. Ginkgo: Fountain of Youth and Vitality

Balon R. *Ginkgo biloba* for antidepressant-induced sexual dysfunction? [letter]. *Journal of Sex and Marital Therapy*, 1999, *25*, 1–10.

Cesarani A, Meloni F, Alpini D, et al. *Ginkgo biloba* (Egb 761) in the treatment of equilibrium disorders. *Adv Ther*, 1998, *15*, 291–304.

Cohen AJ, Bartlik B. *Ginkgo biloba* for antidepressant-induced sexual dysfunction. *Journal of Sex and Marital Therapy*, 1998, *24*, 139–143.

Curtis-Prior P, Vere D, Fray P. Therapeutic value of *Ginkgo biloba* in reducing symptoms of decline in mental function. *Journal of Pharmacy and Pharmacology*, 1999, *51*, 535–541.

Dubreuil C. Therapeutic trial in acute cochlear deafness: A comparative study of *Ginkgo biloba* extract and nicergoline [In French]. *La Presse Médicale*, 1986, *15*, 1559–1561.

Emerit I, Arutyunyan R, Oganesian N, et al. Radiation-induced clastogenic factors: Anticlastogenic effect of *Ginkgo biloba* extract. *Free Radical Biology and Medicine*, 1995, *18*, 985–991.

Emerit I, Oganesian N, Sarkisian T, et al. Clastogenic factors in the plasma of

Chernobyl accident recovery workers: Anticlastogenic effect of *Ginkgo biloba* extract. *Radiation Research*, 1995, *144*, 198–205.

Geßner B, Voelp A, Klasser M. Study of the long-term action of a *Gingo biloba* extract on vigilance and mental performance as determined by means of quantitative EEG and psychometric measurements [In German]. *Arzneimittelforschung*, 1985, *35*, 1459–1465.

Ginkgo protects against altitude sickness. *Herbalgram*, 1999, *46*, 20.

Haguenauer JP, Cantenot F, Koskas H, et al. Treatment of equilibrium disorders with *Ginkgo biloba* extract: A multicenter double-blind drug versus placebo study [In French]. *La Presse Médicale*, 1986, *15*, 1569–1572.

Halpern G. *Ginkgo: A practical guide*. Garden City Park, NY: Avery, 1998.

Hindmarch I. Activity of *Ginkgo biloba* extract on short-term memory [In French]. *La Presse Médicale*, 1986, *15*, 1592–1594.

Hopfenmuller W. Nachweis der therapeutischen Wirsamkeit eines *Ginkgo biloba*-Spezialextraktes: Meta-Analyse von 11 klinischen Studien bei Patienten mit Hirnleistungsstorungen im Alter. *Arzneimittelforschung*, 1994, *44*, 1005–1013.

Itil TM, Eralp E, Tsambis E, et al. Central nervous system effects of *Ginkgo biloba*, a plant extract. *American Journal of Therapeutics*, 1996, *3*, 63–73.

Jung F, Mrowietz C, Kiesewetter H, et al. Effect of *Ginkgo biloba* on fluidity of blood and peripheral microcirculation in volunteers [In German]. *Arzneimittelforschung*, 1990, *40*, 589–593.

Kanowski S, Herrmann WM, Stephan K, et al. Proof of efficacy of the GB special extract Egb 761 in outpatients suffering from mild to moderate primary degenerative dementia of the Alzheimer type or multi-infarct dementia. *Phytomedicine*, 1997, *4*, 3–13.

Kleijnen J, Knipschild P. *Ginkgo biloba* for cerebral insufficiency. *British Journal of Clinical Pharmacy*, 1992, *34*, 352–358.

Lanthony P, Cosson JP. The course of color vision in early diabetic retinopathy treated with *Ginkgo biloba* extract: A preliminary double-blind versus placebo study [In French]. *Journal Francais de Ophthalmologie*, 1988, *11*, 671–674.

LeBars PL, Katz MM, Berman N, et al. A placebo-controlled, double-blind, randomized trial of an extract of GB for dementia. *Journal of the American Medical Association*, 1997, *278*, 1327–1332.

Lebuisson DA, Leroy L, Rigal G. Treatment of senile macular degeneration with *Ginkgo biloba* extract: A preliminary double-blind drug versus placebo study [In French]. *La Presse Médicale*, 1986, *15*, 1556–1558.

Matthews MK, Jr. Association of GB with intracerebral hemorrhage [letter]. *Neurology*, 1998, *50*, 1933–1934.

Meyer B. Multicenter randomized double-bind drug versus placebo study of the treatment of tinnitus with *Ginkgo biloba* extract [In French]. *La Presse Médicale*, 1986, *15*, 1562–1564.

Oken BS, Storzbach DM, Kaye JA. The efficacy of GB on cognitive function in Alzheimer's disease. *Archives of Neurology*, 1998, *55*, 1409–1415.

Perry E, Pickering AT, Wang EE, et al. Medicinal plants and Alzheimer's disease: From ethnobotany to phytotherapy. *Journal of Pharmacy and Pharmacology*, 1999, *510*, 527–534.

Peters H, Kieser M, Holscher U. Demonstration of the efficacy of GB special extract EGb 671 on intermittent claudication: A placebo-controlled, double-blind multicenter trial. *Vasa*, 1998, *27*, 106–110.

Pietri S, Seguin JR, d'Arbigny P, et al. *Ginkgo biloba* extract (Egb 761) pretreatment limits free radical-induced oxidative stress in patients undergoing coronary bypass surgery. *Cardiovascular Drug Therapy*, 1997, *11*, 121–131.

Pietschmann A, Kuklinski B, Otterstein A. Protection from UV-light-induced oxidative stress by nutritional radical scavengers [In German]. *Zeitschrift für Gesamte Inn Med*, 1992, *47*, 518–522.

Raabe A, Raabe M, Ihm P. Therapeutic follow-up using automatic perimetry in chronic cerebroretinal ischemia in elderly patients: Prospective double-blind study with graduated dose *Ginkgo biloba* treatment [In German]. *Klinische Monatsblaetter für Augenheilkunde*, 1991, *199*, 432–438.

Rai GS, Shovlin C, Wesnes KA. A double-bind placebo controlled study of *Ginkgo biloba* extract ("tanakan") in elderly outpatients with mild to moderate memory impairment. *Current Research and Medical Opinion*, 1991, *12*, 350–355.

Rigney U, Kimber S, Hindmarch I. The effects of acute doses of standardized *Ginkgo biloba* extract on memory and psychomotor performance in volunteers. *Phytotherapy Research*, 1999, *13*, 408–415.

Roncin JP, Schwartz F, De'Arbigby P. Egb 761 in control of acute mountain sickness and vascular reactivity to cold exposure. *Aviation Space Environmental Medicine*, 1996, *67*, 445–452.

Schneider B. *Ginkgo biloba* extract in peripheral arterial diseases: Meta-analysis of controlled clinical studies [In German]. *Arzneimittelforschung*, 1992, *42*, 428–436.

Skogh M. Extracts of GB and bleeding or haemorrhage. *Lancet*, 1998, *352*, 1145–1146.

Skolnick A. Old Chinese herbal medicine used for fever yields possible new Alzheimer disease therapy. *Journal of the American Medical Association*, 1997, *227*, 776

Vale S. Subarachnoid hemorrhage associated with *Ginkgo biloba*. *Lancet*, 1998, *352*(9121), 36.

Van Beek TA, Bombardelli E, Morazzoni P, et al. *Ginkgo biloba* L. *Fitoterapia*, 1998, *49*, 195–244.

Warot D, Lacomblez L, Danjou P, et al. Comparative effects of *Ginkgo biloba* extracts on psychomotor performances and memory in healthy subjects. *Therapie*, 1991, *46*, 33–36.

Witte S, Anadere I, Walitza E. Improvement of hemorherology with *Ginkgo biloba* extract: Decreasing a cardiovascular risk factor [In German]. *Fortschritte Medizin*, 1992, *110*, 247–250.

CHAPTER 4. Valerian: Nature's Sandman

Albrecht M, Berger W, Laux P, et al. Psychopharmaceuticals and safety in traffic [In German]. *Zeitschrift fur Allgemeinmedizin*, 1995, *71*, 1215–1221.

Andeatini R, Leite JR. Effect of valepotriates on the behavior of rats in the elevated plus-maze during diazepam withdrawal. *European Journal of Pharmacology*, 1994, *260*, 233–235.

Balderer G, Borbely AA. Effect of valerian on human sleep. Psychopharmacology, 1985, *87*, 406–409.

Bos R, Hendriks H, Scheffer JJC, Woerdenbag HJ. Cytotoxic potential of valerian constituents and valerian tinctures. *Phytomedicine*, 1998, *5*, 219–225.

Bos R, Woerdenbag HJ, Hendriks H, et al. Analytical aspects of phytotherapeutic valerian preparations. *Phytochemical Analysis*, 1996, *7*, 143–151.

Bos R, Woerdenbag HJ, van Putten FMS, et al. Seasonal variation of the essential oil, valerenic acid and derivatives, and valepotriates in *Valleriana officinalis* roots and rhizomes, and the selection of plants suitable for phytomedicines. *Planta Medica*, 1998, *64*, 143–147.

Bounthanh C, Bergmann C, Beck JP, et al. Valepotriates: A new class of cytotoxic and antitumor agents. *Planta Medica*, 1981, *41*, 21–28.

Bourin M, Bougerol T, Guitton B, et al. A combination of plant extracts in the treatment of outpatient with adjustment disorder with anxious mood: Controlled study versus placebo. *Fundamentals of Clinical Pharmacology*, 1997, *11*, 127–132.

British Herbal Pharmacopoeia. Bournemouth, UK: British Herbal Medical Association, 1983.

Brown D. *Herbal Prescriptions for Better Health*. Rocklin, CA: Prima Publishing, 1996.

Chan TYK. An assessment of the delayed effects associated with valerian overdose [Letter]. *International Journal of Clinical Pharmacology and Therapeutics*, 1998, *36*, 569.

Culpeper, N. (1953) *Culpeper's Complete Herbal: A book of Natural Remedies for Ancient Ills*. London: Wordsworth Reference Editions, 1995.

Donath F, Bravo SQ, Diefenbach I, et al. Polysomnographic and subjective findings in insomniacs under treatment with placebo and valerian extract (LI 156). *Proceedings of the 2nd International Congress on Phytomedicine*, Munich, Germany, 1996.

European Pharmacopeia. 2nd ed. St. Ruffine, France: Maissonneuvre, 1985.

Garges HP, Varia I, Doraiswamy PM. Cardiac complications and delirium associated with valerian root withdrawal [letter]. *Journal of the American Medical Association*, 1998, *280*, 1566–1567.

Gerard, J. (1597) *Gerard's Herbal*. Edited by Marcus Woodward. London: Studio Editions, 1990.

Gerhard U, Hobi V, Kocher R, et al. Acute sedative effect of a herbal relaxation tablet as compared to that of bromazepam [In German]. *Schweizerische Rundschau für Medizin Praxis*, 1996, *80*, 1481–1486.

Gerhard U, Linnenbrink N, Georghiadou C, et al. Vigilence-decreasing effects of 2 plant-derived sedatives [In German]. *Schweizerische Rundschau für Medizin Praxis*, 1996, *85*, 473–481.

Hansel R, Schulz J. GABA and other amino acids in Valerian root [In German]. *Archiv der Pharmazie*, 1981, *314*, 380–381.

Hendriks H, Bos R, Woerdenbag HJ, et al. Central nervous system depressant activity of valerenic acid in the mouse. *Planta Medica*, 1985, *51*, 28–31.

Hobbs C. *Valerian: The Relaxing and Sleep Herb*. Capitola, CA: Botanica Press, 1994.

Houghton PJ. (Ed.). *Valerian: The Genus Valeriana*. The Netherlands: Harwood Academic Publishers, 1997.

Houghton PJ. The biological activity of valerian and related plants. *Journal of Ethnopharmacology*, 1998, *22*, 121–142.

Jansen W. Doppelblindstudie mit Baldrisedon. *Therapiewoche*, 1977, *27*, 2779–2786.

Kamm-Kohl AV, Jansen W, Brockmann P. Modern valerian therapy of nervous disorders in elderly patients. *Medwelt*, 1984, *35*, 1450–1454.

Kohnen R, Oswald WD. The effects of valerian, propranolol, and their combination on activation, performance, and mood of healthy volunteers under social stress conditions. *Pharmacopsychiatry*, 1988, *21*, 447–448.

Leathwood PD, Chauffard F. Quantifying the effect of mild sedatives. *Journal of Psychiatric Research*, 1983, *17*, 115–122.

Leathwood PD, Chauffard F. Aqueous extract of valerian reduce latency to fall asleep in man. *Planta Medica*, 1984, *51*, 144–148.

Leathwood PD, Chauffard F, Heck E, et al. Aqueous extract of valerian root (*Valeriana officinalis* L.) improves sleep quality in man. *Pharmacology, Biochemistry and Behavior*, 1982, *17*, 65–71.

Leathwood PD, Chauffard F, Munoz-Box R. *The effects of valerian on subjective and objective sleep parameters*. Poster presented at 6th European Congress of Sleep Research, Zurich, 1982.

Lindahl O, Lindwall L. Double-blind study of a valerian preparation. *Pharmacology, Biochemistry, and Behavior*, 1989, *32*, 1065–1066.

Lutkowski J, Turowska M. Effect of relative humidity on the content of valepotriates and volatile oil in *Valeriana officinalis*. *Herba Polonica*, 1973, *19*, 338–341.

Macgregor FB, Abernathy VE, Dahabra S, et al. Hepatoxicity of herbal remedies. *British Medical Journal*, 1989, *299*, 1156–1157.

Martindale. *The Extra Pharmacopoeia*. 22nd ed. London: Pharmaceutical Press, 1941.

Morin CM, Colecchi C, Stone J, et al. Behavioral and pharmacological therapies for late-life insomnia: A randomized controlled trial. *Journal of the American Medical Association*, 1999, *281*, 991–999.

Moser L. Arzneimittel bei stress am steuer? *Deutsche Apotheker Zeitung*, 1981, *121*, 2651–2654.

Murray MT. *The Healing Power of Herbs*. 2nd ed. Rocklin, CA: Prima Publishing, 1995.

Newall CA, Anderson LA, Phillipson JD. *Herbal Medicines: A Guide for Health-Care Professionals*. London: Pharmaceutical Press, 1996.

Oshima Y, Matsukoka S, Ohizumi Y. Antidepressant principles of *Valeriana fauriei* roots. *Chemical and Pharmaceutical Bulletin*, 1995, *43*, 169–170.

Riedel E, Hansel R, Ehrke G. Inhibition of gamma-aminobutyric acid catabolism by valerenic acid derivatives. *Planta Medica*, 1982, *46*, 219–220.

Rosencrans JA, Defeo JJ, Youngken HW. Pharmacological investigation of certain *Valeriana officnalis* L. extracts. *Journal of Pharmaceutical Sciences*, 1961, *50*, 240–244.

Sakamoto T, Mitani Y, Nakajima K. Psychotropic effects of Japanese valerian root extract. *Chemical and Pharmaceutical Bulletin*, 1992, *40*, 758–761.

Samuelsson G. *Drugs of Natural Origin: A Textbook of Pharmacognosy*. Stockholm: Swedish Pharmaceutical Press, 1992.

Santos MS, Ferreira F, Faro C, et al. The amount of GABA present in aqueous extracts of valerian is sufficient to account for [^{3}H]GABA release in synaptosomes. *Planta Medica*, 1994, *60*, 475–476.

Schulz H, Jobert M. Die darstellung sedierender/tranquilisierender wirkungen von phytopharmaka im quantifizierten EEG [abstract]. *Zeitschrift für Phytotherapie Abstractband*, 1995, p. 10.

Schulz H, Stolz C, Muller J. The effect of valerian extract on sleep polygraphy in poor sleepers: A pilot study. *Pharmacopsychiatry*, 1994, *27*, 147–151.

Schulz V, Hansel R, Tyler V. *Rational Phytotherapy: A Physician's Guide to Herbal Medicine*. 3rd ed. Berlin: Springer-Verlag, 1998.

Scudder JM. *Specific Medications and Specific Medicine*. Cincinnati: Scudder Brothers, 1903.

Stahl E, Schild W. Uber die Verbreitung der aquilibrierend wirkenden valepotriate in der familie der *Valerinaceae*. *Phytochemistry*, 1971, *10*, 147–153.

Steinegger E, Hansel R. *Textbook of Pharmacognosy and Phytopharmacology*. 4th ed. Berlin: Springer-Verlag, 1979.

Stoll A, Seececk E, Stauffacher D. New investigations on valerian [In German]. *Schweizerische Apotheker Zeitung*, 1957, *95*, 115–120.

Stuart M. (Ed.). *The Encyclopedia of Herbs and Herbalism.* New York: Crescent Books, 1979.

Tufik S, Fujita K, deLourdes V, et al. Effects of a prolonged administration of valepotriates in rats on the mothers and their offspring. *Journal of Ethnopharmacology,* 1994, *41*, 39–44.

Upton R, Barrett M, Williamson E, et al. *Valerian Root, Valeriana Officinalis: Analytical Quality Control and Therapeutic Monograph.* Santa Cruz, CA: American Herbal Pharmacopoeia, 1999.

von Eikstedt KW. Die reeinflussung der alkohol-wirkung durch valepotriate. *Arnzeimittelforschung,* 1969, *19*, 995–997.

Vorbach EU, Gortelmayer R, Bruning J. Therapie von insomnien: Wirksamkeit und vertraglichkeit eines Baldrian-Praparates. *Psychopharmakotherapie,* 1996, *3*, 109–115.

Willey LB, Mady SP, Cobaugh DJ, et al. Valerian overdose: A case report. *Veterinary and Human Toxicology,* 1995, *37*, 364–365.

Index

About
the Authors

Jonathan R. T. Davidson, MD, is a professor in the department of psychiatry and behavioral sciences at Duke University Medical Center in Durham, North Carolina, where he is also Director of the Anxiety and Traumatic Stress Program. He earned his medical degree at University College and University College Hospital Medical School in London. In addition to board certification in psychiatry in the United States, he is also a Fellow of the American Psychiatric Association, the Royal College of Psychiatrists (United Kingdom) and the American College of Neuropsychopharmacology. He has conducted many treatment outcome studies that evaluated medicines or psychotherapy in schizophrenia, depression, traumatic stress, and anxiety. He has received several grants from the National Institutes of Health, and has served as chairman of the NIMH Treatment Assessment Review Committee. He serves on the board of directors of the Anxiety Disorders Association of America. He was also co-chair of the American Psychiatric Association's DSM-IV Work Group for posttraumatic stress disorder (PTSD). He has authored two books on PTSD and social phobia. He has, in addition, published over 200 papers and 50 chapters. He is actively involved in research in complementary and alternative treatments and received professional training in homeopathic medicine in the United Kingdom.

Kathryn M. Connor, MD, is a graduate of the University of Maryland School of Medicine in Baltimore. She completed her residency training in psychiatry at Duke University Medical Center in Durham, North Carolina, followed by a research fellowship in clinical psychopharmacology at Glaxo Wellcome in Research Triangle Park, North Carolina, and Duke University. She has continued on the Duke faculty as an assistant professor in the department of psychiatry and behavioral sciences and is the research director of the Anxiety and Traumatic Stress Program at Duke. In addition to a clinical practice, she is involved in clinical research in anxiety and mood disorders, and is a principal or co-investigator in a variety of studies, including treatment trials of medications, herbs, and other therapies. She has published numerous scientific papers, has presented at major national and international professional meetings, and recently authored a book on Kava, *Kava: Nature's Stress Relief.* Dr. Connor has received a number of awards in recognition of her work. She is also a member of the Data Safety Monitoring Board for the National Center for Complementary and Alternative Medicine at the National Institutes of Health.

DISCARD